Happiness: The Yoga Power of Rehearsal

Moving Life Forward with Intended Purpose

Dr. Bryan Silva, Ph.D.

Making sense of things that have transpired in your life while avoiding the depression, anxiety, and desperation pitfalls that lurk within all of us.

Happiness: The Yoga Power of Rehearsal
Copyright © 2014 by Bryan Silva

ISBN-13: 978-1497409743
ISBN-10: 1497409748

Cover design by: Colleen Krause

DEDICATION

This book is dedicated to my wife and daughters whom I love with all of my heart. The book is also dedicated to all of those special persons and family members who I am proud to call friends. Lastly, I dedicate this book to those persons who will read it and transform their lives into a happiness state that I know is possible for all human beings.

Table of Contents

Foreword

You never know when your life is about to change. While you realize that you are undergoing minor daily changes, the big change often times presents itself in an abrupt manner. The loss of a job, the news about terminal cancer, the presentation of a pending divorce, the ending of a relationship, the death of a family member or friend, are all tragic situations that come unexpectedly. We may believe that we are prepared for each of these situations but this belief is merely imaginary. Personal change takes a calculated commitment and persistent action.

You and I are about to embark on a unique journey. Questions swirl around our minds. 'Was there anything I could have done that could have altered the course of events in my life? Were there any signs or symptoms that I missed or have I failed to act in a different manner just before the life-changing event? If this were possible, would I have taken action?' As humans we all have these after the fact moments. We ponder on the current events and re-hash the past in search for material or bits of information that we could learn from and possibly apply to our future decisions.

If you have ever felt depression, anxiety, confusion, anger, regret, or desperation, you will personally connect with several areas of this book. Some of you are enduring the toughest times of your life as you read this book. Your mind is spinning like a computer's hard drive with no end in sight. You lack sleep. You are tired. You are bothered by thoughts of events that have altered and are altering your life's course. Some of you may be asking: 'How could this have happened to me?' Others may be seeking for an end to the pain and agony that such events have caused in their daily lives.

I can tell you this: Only when you are ready for positive change, will it begin to take root. Only when you choose to abandon the past and begin a new life today will you begin to enjoy the new life that has been waiting for you. Only when you stop rehashing the complicated events that transpired in the past, will your mind be allowed to absorb new and positive memories. Don't live in the past. Our intended purpose reveals itself only after the clouds have cleared.

The most important goal in most humans' lives is to be happy. Yet, to achieve happiness, humans must allow their minds to release the past and move forward into the future with intended purpose. You were rich once and now you are poor. You were poor once and now you are rich. Your future is always half-chanced. Half the time you are on top, and the other half… you may have fallen into disgrace. Sadly, most of these feelings of disgrace are self-made by our own minds. You are the one who is immersed into self-pity. *Once you realize that you are the one who creates your own reality*, this is the very power you need to set yourself free.

Life is a Gift and Staying Focused on what is important requires Personal Rehearsal Strength. As you read this Yoga Power of Rehearsal book, begin to think of the possibilities that are available in your life towards achieving happiness. Life is the most important starting point. *If you are alive, anything is possible.* Whether you are the fastest runner in the world, or a recent paraplegic, positive change is possible. Whether you have sight or are blind, positive change is possible. Yet, the only way for you to become positive and happy is to accept that you are broken and need to be fixed.

The year is 2014. This book is based on my own life's turmoil and lessons learned along the way. I don't propose to know the answers to all of life's questions, yet – *I introduce myself to you as an agent of change.* I have been where you are now and have chosen to offer you simple suggestions that if you act upon them, you will begin to see a change in your life that will attract other positive changes and ultimately bring you a new level of happiness.

Liberate your mind from the unnecessary worrying and suffering. Universal Happiness is possible and it takes one person at a time. You can be that person. This story is all about you and for YOU—Claim your transformation into joyfulness.

Dr. Bryan Silva, Ph.D.

Introduction

Who is that person whom my mind thinks about, worries about, offers advice to? That person is **Me**. I am that person. I know that worrying only results in stress. Yet, I allow it to enter my body continually and remain there as a cancer that only aims to destroy my life. Why do I let it? *Because I haven't been taught not to allow it.*

What am I feeding my mind? Is this food benefiting my soul or degrading my full potential? Am I ready for change? Will I take action towards positive change in my life? The choice has always been mine, yet I accepted the chains and the anchors that simply would not set me free.

Then the day came. The day when I chose not to wear the heavy chains or drag the archaic anchors. *Freedom arrived and I was ready for it.* I had been in pain. I had suffered enough. That day was the day where I wouldn't look back. That day was the day where I chose to live my life the way it was meant to be lived.

The purpose of this book is to bring you into a place of peacefulness, contentment, and happiness. *Living a better life that is full of prosperity and freedom is possible.* If you have been feeling down lately or during those times when you are feeling down, pick up this book and open it up to any section of your choosing. Advice in this book is aimed at repairing your internal being. However, the only way this repair can happen is for you to wipe clean your belief systems and other anchors that have made you a prisoner for so long. *Free up your mind so that the right thoughts and feelings will begin to flow throughout your mind and body.* Do listen to the advice in this book but find those very pieces that will bring you into a happy state in your own life.

What this book is. This book is not a chronological order of events. Instead, it is about life advice that you can tailor to your specific needs. This book is not about yoga physical exercise but rather about repetitive yoga mental exercises. Rather than a storyline, information in this book jumps back and forth in thought as a way to rattle your current thinking process and to stimulate your desire for positive change.

Information in this book is aimed at disciplining your mind to achieve that which you never thought possible. The mind is the body's central command center. Learn to disconnect from your worries and you will put your mind's power to work on instant focus and clarity. Learn to control your mind and find that you will be able to clear out the distractions that have been keeping you back for far too long. Master this yoga rehearsal process and see the impossible become the possible.

Living in a happy state in one's life brings not only happiness but health, well-being, and mind liberation. Opportunities that you never knew existed present themselves and you will ask: *Where were these before?* The simple answer is that we attract what we become. If you were sad, depressed, angry, confused, overwhelmed, anxious, or discouraged you were not ready for this complete change. Now that you have suffered, or experienced loss, or reflected, and/or endured tremendous pain, you are ready for this Yoga Power of Rehearsal transformation. Allow no one to stop that which you were intended to accomplish on this earth. This is your life and this is your body.

Write your own story. Find that place which validates you as a human being. Once you arrive, take it all in. Plan every action towards staying there.

Chapter 1: The Yoga Power of Rehearsal

Human beings are unlike any other animal on earth. We are intelligent creatures who are constantly learning. We learn from personal mistakes and from positive actions. We learn from others' mistakes and from watching events unfold. We make decisions on whether we would like or would not like to participate in certain events. Who we decide to embrace as friends often highly depends on what "vibe" they project as we are introduced to them. We find that "chemistry" whether perceived or real, is what drives us to befriend or push away others.

As intelligent human beings we also have the Yoga Power of Rehearsal. I have labeled it the Yoga power of rehearsal as, similar to Yoga, we already have the ability to make ourselves happy without any additional pieces other than what has been provided in our minds. You agree that we have the power to dream. Such power also provides us with the ability to rehearse upcoming decisions in our minds. Without any money, we can close our eyes and place our presence within any scenario we choose. In our minds we have the power to glamorize ourselves or to belittle our existence.

Liberate Your Mind

In Hindu philosophy, Yoga is defined as a practice that teaches people to experience inner peace. Such peace can only be achieved once one controls their mind and body. Yet, to control your mind, you must clear out the clutter and liberate it from the normal and everyday worries. *You and only you – must learn to suppress or re-route those thoughts,* which are hindering your ability to become happy or happier.

This liberation process will happen only after you have rehearsed a number of positive exercises aimed at clearing your mind from the distractions. You must know that your physical and mental well-being is directly connected to what your mind is thinking and feeling on a daily basis. Feed your mind positive thoughts and discipline it to push away negative thoughts and feelings. *Yes it can be done. Yes, it will be done.* But, it will take some yoga rehearsal power with personal intention and direct actions on your part to make it a reality.

Happiness requires not only a liberation of the mind but your ability to *become selfish on your own personal happiness. Take a break from helping others.* Today you must and will put yourself first in order to become happy. Read this book's recipe and follow it by gathering all the necessary ingredients.

Happiness requires your immediate attention. Happiness will bring you to a new and improved level of positive mental and physical well-being status. Allow your mind to accept this new philosophy and begin living today the way your life was meant to be lived.

We hold the Power to Change

Unbeknownst to many, we actually have the power to decide where our dreams will take us and what outcomes each of these journeys will present. You will be surprised that we can actually rehearse any situation in our minds that allows us to simulate separate conclusions. Try this. Close your eyes and ponder how you would feel if you were completely poor, living under a cold bridge or you are extremely rich, living in the most beautiful home with a beautiful and healthy family.

As you read this book, some of you will allow these ideas and positive thoughts to enter your mind while others, who maybe a bit skeptical are denying any permission for new thoughts to enter their minds. Such skepticism is often attributed to the amount of major life traumas that you have experienced in your life. If your life has been for the most part without turmoil, you may be more open to my positive ideas in this book and will actually allow your mind to absorb this information without much hesitation. However, if your life has involved a number of challenges that can be labeled as turmoil, these may actually hinder the ability of your mind to move to a happier place.

Moving to a state of Yoga Rehearsal mode demands that if it has been at least three months since the incident has happened, it will have no impact on your overall happiness.

Stop re-living tragic events

Stop re-living the tragic event. Stop playing the same record over and over in your head. Begin to practice rehearsing positive scenarios in your mind. You can start small: Close your eyes. You are a young child visiting a large clothing store with your parents when you get lost inside the store. You desperately search each section of the store – scared that something may happen to you when suddenly, you hear your mom say: "There you are!" As your mom extends her hand, you grab it and immediately give her a big hug. You are safe now. You feel warm all over. As you embrace your parent your fears have suddenly vanished. Safety is often the start of happiness.

Let's take another situation: Close your eyes and sit down. Ignore the noises. Block out all distractions. You are hungry and have not eaten for quite some time. Your stomach aches and you are confident that this pain stems from lack of food. You have tried to beg for some money but people have simply ignored your verbal requests. You are sad. You just wish that you could eat anything to improve your survival ability. You feel tired and defeated. Suddenly, without any explanation, a family stops by you and hands you a warm package. You can smell that it is fresh food. As you open the package, you find that it is wonderfully looking fresh food. You thank them from the bottom of your heart. As you begin to eat the food, you realize how wonderful and fresh it tastes. It is the best food you have tasted in a long time. You take your time eating this food – chewing slowly as a way to taste the flavor and aroma that has now consumed your moment. You learn from this experience that nutrition is important to happiness. If you are hungry, you often feel defeated. Once you eat, the body thanks you. This action is in fact happiness.

Small Accomplishments

Small accomplishments, each at different levels and intervals, do in fact bring you happiness. Overall happiness is built in small steps. Each time you perform an action that brings you a certain amount of happiness it proves to you that happiness is in fact a possibility. Just as important to achieving happiness is the fact that once you perform an action that brings you sadness, you will need to learn to avoid performing such action again. It will take some discipline and possible sacrifices to avoid making the same mistakes twice *but, it can be done.* Others have done it and you too can do it.

Ignore the Nay-Sayers

Do not waste a single second worrying or thinking about those people who did not help you at a time of need. Instead, embrace and love those people who were there for you during those times of need.

Every time we as humans want to do something to better our lives, there will be those who will tell us that: "No, it can't be done" or, "Others have tried that before and failed so you shouldn't try it." We label these "No" people as nay-sayers. Every time you want to make a positive change in your life those nay-sayers will simply disagree that *it can be done.* Some people will actually spend more time trying to explain to you why a new change will not work versus trying to see how it can work. *You must label these people nay-sayers and make a conscious effort to ignore them.* They are wasteful distractions. Successful large and innovative corporations have learned all about these negative people and you should too.

A new trending idea presents itself and your excited about the change. You research the possibilities and see that these are real. You speak with others and through research obtain real evidence that this new idea is possible and would bring wealth to you and your family. Once this happens, ask yourself if your body wants it. Close your eyes and ask it in a quiet environment if this is what you should do. The answer will present itself. Follow that answer. Do what is necessary and put the right amount of action behind this new idea. Know this: *Every day others become successful and you can too.* Today is your turn.

Read non-fiction books. Read about both sides of any topic. Read as much as you can on any trending topic. Become an expert on that trending topic. Others will then want to listen to what you have to say about the topic. All of this is possible only if you ignore the nay-sayers and stop worrying about other people who don't really matter in your life.

Minimize your worst possible outcome. If you are participating in risky behavior, continuing such behavior will only get you one step closer to disaster. Once disaster arrives, only those who are resilient will survive the strong winds and roll-a-coaster of emotions associated with such collision and loss. You can avoid the storm. It is never too late to set a new course. Pay attention to advice given in this book if you wish to get on the right track of living the righteous **Life**.

Chapter 2: Believe in the Now

The best way towards achieving happiness is to expose that which makes you unhappy. Once you expose those very things or issues that make you unhappy, you will need to allow your body and mind to begin a re-configuration process. Such process involves abandoning old beliefs, removing biases, prejudices, and some man-made theories that have kept you away from reality for far too long.

A key difference between those who are truly happy and not so happy is to look at them from various viewpoints. How is it that so many people are happy and you continue to be unhappy? If as you read this book you feel that your life is perfect, then this is not the book for you. However, if you feel that there are pieces missing from your life that you would like to find in order to become happy, then continue reading.

Becoming happy takes some work and requires a number of personal sacrifices. The work that I refer to is more in the form of taking action instead of remaining in neutral, blind-eye, or ignorant neutral mode. The sacrifices that I refer to involve removing the artificial anchors that have kept you in the same place for far too long. It is time to wipe your mind clean and allow new thoughts, ideas, and beliefs to enter and bring you natural happiness.

Stop living in the past! Stop rehashing past events. Stop allowing fear and ignorance to prevent you from arriving at a place of peacefulness. Stop listening to the media while hoping that somehow it will make you a better person. Begin opening up your eyes to new possibilities. Begin feeling how great it is to be alive. Look around at this huge world that you use to call a playground when you were younger. Find the child in you. Allow that child to play uninterrupted.

Live in the present. Abandon the past. I realize that you may have lots of prior stories to tell but this very moment is yours to shape. Take this moment to learn about the Yoga Power of Rehearsal and how it can *reprogram your mind to accept the positive that is abundant on this earth.* If you accept that any life-changing event is based on perspective, then you will be successful in arriving at a more peaceful place than where you are at this very moment.

Turn off your smart phone. Turn off your cell phone. Turn off the TV. Turn off the Internet. Turn off the computer. Turn off the music radio. Turn off all possible sounds and listen. Allow your mind to be okay with quietness and stillness. You need this experience in order to allow your mind to expand. It may be uncomfortable at first, but you can do it. You have the power to do it. Release that power. Take control of your mind and watch how arriving at a place of happiness will completely change your life for the positive.

Never give up. No matter what you are facing. *Know this:* Everybody, no matter how they look on the outside, are also having real issues on the inside that they are continually dealing with. *This applies to everyone.* It doesn't matter if the person is good looking, or not. It doesn't matter if the person is successful, or not. It doesn't matter if they have a job, or money, or a beach house, or a nice car. Everyone means everyone in the basic sense of the word.

Worries

Human beings worry about... well, things. Some of these worries
are minor and other ones tend to overwhelm our minds. *The
reality is that most of these worries never happen.* If they do
happen, many of the worries are never as severe as human
beings projected them to be. Worrying is then part of human
protocol. Yet, many must know that worrying will not change
the course of what is going to happen anyway.
Do you need help learning not to worry? Read and memorize
the *Serenity Prayer.* Say it to yourself each time your worries are
trying to consume your mind.

God grant me the serenity to accept the things I cannot
change, the courage to change the things I can, and the
wisdom to know the difference.

Anonymous

Balloon Experiment

A small child attaches an empty balloon to the end of a running
water hose. As the water enters the opening, the balloon begins
to expand. You watch the balloon knowing full well that it will
eventually explode. You know that the balloon has its limitations.
You have possibly seen this experiment before. You know what
is about to happen, yet -- you worry. You cringe knowing that at
any moment the balloon will explode and water will be
everywhere. Finally, it happens. The balloon explodes and the
person who was filling it, almost didn't expect that it would
happen as it did. The reality is that if we are distracted, events
happen around us in *'surprise'* mode. At the same time, some
people are obsessed at looking at the balloon and waiting for the
second when it will explode.

The balloon actually signifies an event in our lives. It could be a positive or negative event. Yet, the anticipation feeling is very similar to what I just described to you. You become anxious. You worry that the balloon will rip and burst. You wonder when will it break? When it does, you wonder if you and others around you are prepared for it. And, you know what? Once the balloon bursts and water is everywhere, you look around and realize that you and others are okay. The entire experience made you a stronger person without you even realizing it. Now...after this explanation you will be prepared for the next balloon experience. You will find that although you may be frightened, the next time a similar event happens, you won't be as surprised. Chaos may then be acceptable to a certain extent.

The reality in our lives is that the abnormal at times becomes the normal and events that you did not feel would be welcomed, at times become acceptable and somewhat familiar. This applies to all life events including relationships, friendships, marriages, divorces, loss of a job or jobs, loss of home, loss of family or friends, and surprise illnesses.

The happiness reality ingredient is that we have to believe in the Now. The past has passed and there are no guarantees in anyone's future. As you endure what you are enduring now, others are enduring similar and even worse experiences. If they are successful in dealing with their obstacles, you should take notice. However, if they are not successful in dealing with their conflict, personal loss, negative emotions, friendships, and responsibilities, you should not take notice other than to learn what not to do. Learn from others' mistakes. Try to not duplicate others' mistakes.

Theory of Relativity

Remember that in life all is relative. By that I mean that each person's experience may be the worst experience they have ever endured or are enduring in their personal lives. To them, their situation is the direst at the very time they are dealing with it.

They look at other persons who may be going through a tougher situation and still feel that their situation is most serious... because it is. "To each his own" also applies to the tough times we endure in our lives. Each situation brings with it unique components that are directly relative to that person's plight. If you are the person undergoing this "plight," accept the theory of relativity as it will help you eventually solve your situation, or at a minimum, help you through your pain.

Transitions

Everyday of your life you and others are going through transitions. You are changing everyday. Others are changing everyday as well. If you accept this very concept, then you can begin to understand why relationships may at times fail. *If people are changing everyday and you fail to change with the times, you will be left behind.* Those who are left behind oftentimes miss out on what is happening around them. You loved someone so much, yet you failed to recognize that they were going through serious transitions. These transitions changed that person and now he or she no longer loves you. How could this be? All people are continually looking for that which makes them happy. If they are unhappy in a relationship, they will seek other relationships, which can make them happy. If they are unhappy at a job, they will seek out other job opportunities. If they are tired of eating the same food, they will crave for and eventually change the foods they eat.

It is important to pay attention to transitions. Such transitions change the types of clothing styles people like to wear. For example, a person who only wears clothing that was popular in the 1940s may find that it is hard to be accepted in the year 2014. A person who is afraid to kiss their loved one in public may have challenges to overcome if their significant other likes and wants to hug and kiss in public.

Pay special attention to transitions as you live your life. Embrace transitions and allow your body and mind to transform with the changing times.

Society is Cruel

"Normal" often depends on how you fit in. Society is cruel. Whenever you are different, others notice you on a regular basis. You might be what others see, but you don't necessarily have to accept what others see. The decision to be who you are will always rest with you as an individual. *Life is a journey and all of us will endure transitions that will take us to both upper and lower places in our lives.*

Think about this: What if there were no mirrors in this world? What if people couldn't see their reflections on water or glass? Or, what if a person who remembers how great they looked at a certain age lost the ability to use a mirror or to see their reflection? The person would remember how they used to look like on the last time they were able to look into a mirror. So, why the mirror example? Well, *we are our own worst critics.* We see ourselves and always pick out something that could be better. Your hair, your eyes, your face, your body, your hands, your wrinkles, your legs or your mind. You may at times ask yourself: How come I could not look like him or her? Why don't I have good looks or why can't I look like that model?

Read scholarly academic research and you will learn that before they are published, most persons' pictures in model magazines have been touched up an average of thirty times by a digital enhancing computer program such as Photoshop. Their necks can be made to look skinnier, longer, tanned. Blemishes are removed. Cheeks are enhanced to look healthier. Foreheads are extended or compressed. Lips are touched up and enhanced. Eyes are moved up and down according to where they look best within the person's face. The face can be made to look thinner. The people's faces you see in those magazines do not actually exist. No makeup in the entire world, no amount of plastic surgery of any kind... will ever make you look like that picture. If you accept that the picture is not real, then you begin to accept who you are as a person. *You are real.* You are the maker of your own destiny. Stop trying to live in others' shoes. Stop trying to be like others. Like yourself first and the rest will fall into place. Stop or avoid reading beauty magazines. They will damage your mind and distort your perception of the real world.

Everyone is always judging you. Our lives include those who want to help us, those who want to influence us, and those who want us to be like them. Yes, I wrote that correctly, many people in this world enjoy the thrill of being able to influence others in a number of strange ways. Being careful with those who want you to be like them applies to those people who capitalize on trying to be like other influential people. Be kind to those who are willing to give you advice, however, make sure you validate the advice that is being given to you with what you have sought to achieve in your life.

> *What makes you wiser in life is not simply the successes...but when you fall down and come back stronger in life.*

If the advice you receive allows you to *reinforce your intended purpose*, then – yes, listen and take action. However, if the advice you are being given is extreme and goes against your intended life purpose, you must walk away from such anti-growth journey. You must believe that you have been given a Godly intended purpose. God has given you a gift with your life. Treasure this gift. *Grow each day.* Appreciate your gift in a positive way. Push away negativity. Work towards attracting positivity – both in language and in your personal actions.

How are you doing?

The question: "How are you doing" is not a free pass or invitation to tell the next person about your back pain, shoulder pain, neck pain, stomach pain, headaches, and every other negative aspect of your life that you are dealing with. Complaining about all of these at every opportunity will push others away. Others will label you a complainer. Others will shy away from you and avoid asking you how you are doing or feeling. Instead of the complainer attitude, you can answer something like: *"Doing okay. Dealing with some life issues, but you know what? It is great to be alive. It was great seeing you. You look great!"*

Learn the Yoga Power of Rehearsal techniques and motivate yourself each and every day, every single hour of the day. *Don't live your life by default.* You must arrive at a point in time to move forward with intended positive purpose. Understand that it is normal to be or feel a little misguided in life. What is not normal is to allow this misguidance to overwhelm your life, your actions, your dreams, and your desires.

When you find that thing which brings you happiness, embrace it, feed it, and treasure it. Happiness is an event that should be practiced and implemented daily.

Program your mind to be precise on what you desire. Ignore the news – stop watching junk. Stop immersing yourself into TV news and TV shows that influence, and eventually infect your mind. Instead – focus your intentions and desires on living life to its fullest.

Get out and walk. Get out of the house or apartment, or room and see the world. Visit new places. Meet new people. Change your ways – so that you can find out what an amazing gift, the creation of life is. You need to find out who you are without distractions. You have to believe that you were put on this earth for a purpose and to make a difference. *You matter. Your actions matter. Your thoughts matter.* But, – first, these have to matter to you. YES – you must please yourself first before you will be able to please others. Improve yourself first – before you will be able to improve others.

Don't waste time worrying about the things that you cannot control

Look at yourself and if there are things that you don't like in your life, change them. If you are overweight, lose weight. If you are too skinny, eat right so you can gain weight. If you are too weak, take vitamins and eat right. If you are out of shape, exercise. Walking is free.

Now, all of this can only happen by ACTION. Yes, and you know what else? Your history is not your destiny. Stop living in the past. Ignore the past and don't dwell on regrets. **Listen to me:** *Regrets are a waste of human life.* You have a life clock. We are all here on earth for a set number of hours. The more you rehash the past, the more you are burning up valuable life hours.

As you read this advice, you may be thinking: But, But... I like it when people feel sorry for me. OK- I feel you and understand your point... but you are burning up valuable hours to rehash regrets. Such regrets are in the past and cannot be changed. Plus, by rehashing these regrets, you are in fact reinforcing negative energy.

You attract what you believe and if what you believe is that you need to rehash negative experiences over and over, you will become a negative person.

Life is too short to be negative. *You attract people into your life because you are positive energy.* You push people away when you display negative energy. The choice is yours.

Spin your life around. *Do one thing each day that is new and daring.* Get out of your daily routine. Drive a new road on your way to work. If possible, eat at a new healthy restaurant as often as possible. You must believe that from the top of your head to the bottom of your feet, you are perfect in every way. However, for this belief to be real, you must first see yourself as a perfect human being.

I am not saying that you are exactly like others. No. I am telling you that you must like who you are or change the things you do not like about yourself. You are a beautiful human being simply because you have life. *Have you ever wondered just how wonderful being alive is?* Do you know that each and every day there are other people who are laying on a hospital bed dying and wishing they had just one more healthy day to live?

You must believe that if you are alive, you must seek out experiences that confirm your existence. Go to the beach. Go to the mountains. Go to a lake. Visit a river. Go to a park. Sit and watch a waterfall. Visit a Mall. Watch a youth football or a soccer match. Watch a baseball game. Watch a basketball game. Go for a walk.

Believe that sometimes in life, you get dealt the hand that you have been dealt but that it is your responsibility to seek out personal success. If success means being happy, then you be happy. If success means to seek out a job, then seek out a job. If success means to meet a friend – seek out a friend. *You must force yourself to live your own reality. You become the things that you attract.* However, before you can dance with the stars, you must take dance lessons. Have you looked for affordable dance lessons? Have you watched a dance show? Have you asked the right questions in your current life that will allow your life to change for the better?

Know this: It takes a certain type of positive mentality to become successful in life. *Success begins with small steps. Every long journey begins with one single step.* You must put your body in line for that first step. God is already in you. He created you, he is in you ... watching... and offering daily advice. But, along with his advice, the devil is also giving you his evil advice. You must ignore the evil advice and focus on the positive advice.

> ### *You must avoid doing the same thing you have been doing and expecting different results.*

If the road you have been following has not taken you to where you want to go, it is time to find a different road. If the path you have walked has not produced intended results, it is time to abandon that path. There are more than one way to arrive at new grounds. Find your way.

Your History is Not Your Destiny

Have you ever arrived at a building and the front door has been blocked with a "detour" sign steering you into a different direction? You went out of your way and took a different path. As you walked around the building, you saw a beautiful garden. Where in the world? You have worked for this company for five years and had no idea that such a beautiful garden existed behind the building. You took a new path and found a new experience. *This unplanned detour caused you to find something that you were not looking for.* So, listen to what happened: Your history is not your destiny. There comes a time when the experience you are enduring takes you to a new meadow, a new valley, a new country or a new city. *Accept that somewhere along the way, you will find yourself as a fish in strange waters.* You

17

have to believe that life throws you several detour signs that may make you feel uncomfortable. Why the detours? Well, because we are all looking for our own intended purpose.

So, what is your potential? What are your passions? What are your desires? What are your possibilities? What are your options? This is your life and this is your body. Who is the captain of your ship? How long will you keep ignoring the fact that you are in charge of your life? How long do you intend to ignore your potential and live your life on auto-pilot? *What are your fears?* Are you tired of fighting your intended purpose? When will your true choices in life become real? When will you shake off the fear and focus on the fact that you are capable of overcoming every odd? Stop living your life based on what happened in the past. Today is the time for change. Yesterday is too late, and tomorrow offers no guarantees.

Every potential in life is real

Opportunity knocks and you must be ready. You must be the one to put some pressure on yourself to be persistent and focused on what your intended purpose is. You were never intended to simply exist. You are a perfect human being who was designed to be exactly what you are. What others may think is awkward, you know it to be your destiny. Understand that you are the one. You are unique, you are special, you are alive. Know and accept that this is the life you were intended to live. And yet, you need to realize that this is not the end but the beginning. *We are all in transition.*

Greatness is hidden inside of you – waiting to come out. You are worthy of the experiences that await you. If what you are doing is not what you want to do, *find what you want to do.* Take a chance and change your life as each day that passes is one less day you have to live on this earth.

The Power of Practice or Rehearsal

Every superstar will tell you that they endured a significant amount of turmoil in their lives before achieving their popularity and success. Basketball players missed hundreds and even thousands of shots before they became experts at making baskets. Rehearsal is the key to disciplining your body for any change. Strong people who became successful are actual experts at denial, at loss, at losing, at overcoming obstacles.

Make your next shot go in!

Fake it until you make it. Believe that you become successful when you accomplish a goal. It could be a small goal, a medium goal, or a large goal. Create small goals and accomplish those first. Then, create medium goals and accomplish those next. Eventually you will be prepared for larger goals. You pick the time you are ready for the next positive stage.

Getting out of depression oftentimes involves accomplishing small and attainable goals. Chapter 6 discusses depression and ways to avoid it or deal with it.

Look at a map near where you live. Are there any parks nearby? Make it a point to visit a new park. This is your goal. Go to that park on a Saturday where young children are playing. Sit and watch these children play at the playground. No worries, no stresses, no regrets. *Children laugh, yell, scream, run after other children, hide, slide, swing, hang, and play. You see them and accept that they have a certain "ignorance" to the rest of the world.* They have no care in the world. When young children are in the playground, they are being themselves. They do not care what the world thinks of them. They enjoy who they are. Well, you must know that there is a small child inside of you who has been tamed.

This child has been told to stop yelling, stop playing, stop laughing, stop hanging on the playground, stop running, stop dreaming, etc. You have greatness in you that maybe has been stifled by others who felt that you needed to conform to passive societal standards. Ask yourself this: *Who created these archaic standards and why am I still following them?* If your parents or upbringing caused you to feel guilty, why are you still feeling guilty? If they caused you to feel fearful, what can you do to change this? How long do you intend to feel like this? Do you want to change? Are you ready to change?

Internal Positive Spirit

Look into your heart and allow that internal positive spirit to become competitive on a daily basis. Life is one big flowing river. *Water moves past places each and every day.* If you swim in the river today, tomorrow – it will have new water. The reality is that life changes constantly and people who are purpose driven, change their lives with it. *You must change who you are so that you can see positive change in your world.* As the captain of your own ship, you are the one who sets the course.

The reality is that we live in a world that is full of opportunities. Our potential as human beings to succeed is actually influenced by the positive and negative experiences that we endure in our daily lives. *Don't be stagnant.* Move around, visit new places, talk to new people, meet new people, *and take detours on purpose.*

Measure yourself when you are working with people. If you look around and feel that each day you work with this group, you feel like you are dying... then- CHANGE IT! The longer you wait to make this change, the less life you will have tomorrow. While some people such as cancer survivors may have a life changing experience, others may see cancer in their lives and seek out change simply because the life they are living is not the life they were intended to live.

Challenge yourself to get out of the norm. Stop watching extreme and unrealistic TV shows. Stop allowing these shows to change your mental state. Nothing must distract you from being or becoming perfect. Stop listening to the radio in your car. Instead, get some positive thinking tapes and begin listening to these tapes. Listen *to Doctor Bruce Lipton, Don Tolman, Dr. Wayne Dyer, and Jim Rohn.* If you have a smartphone, you can access short clips from these great individual authors on Google's YouTube. If you don't have a smart phone, make your way to the library and access YouTube through computers that provide free Internet access at such public locations. If you have the monetary means, sign up for any upcoming positive thinking seminars or conferences by these great individuals.

Begin with the end in mind. If you want to become successful and positive, then begin feeding your mind and body with those ingredients to achieve future positive outcomes. Speak as if you have already accomplished your goals.

Watch what you say on a daily basis

If you tell yourself: "I feel tired," your body intentionally notifies your genes that it is time to rest. If you tell yourself: "I am too fat," you have just made yourself feel negative by feeling unaccepted. If you tell yourself: "I am so out of shape," then you are in fact telling your body that you lack the normal exercise that is needed to remain healthy. Stop saying these negative things. Instead, take positive action. Schedule set times to go to the gym or to walk around the block. Stop being a human vacuum! Stop putting food items in your mouth that you know are bad or unhealthy for you. Stop eating so late. Stop eating at least two hours before going to sleep. Stop drinking soda. Stop smoking. Drink filtered water. Avoid eating products that contain Gluten.

Ride bikes. WALK! Eat healthy! Eat organic fruits! Stop eating junk and fast-food. Change your eating habits! Stop watching so much TV. *LEARN – Yes, learn to talk positive.* Yes, you may know that you are overweight. But… – say: "I feel so good today that it is time to join a gym!" or "Today is the day to begin my diet" instead of "I will wait to begin my diet on Monday!"

Think: Eat foods with Fiber and Celebrate the small wins! Today you lost one pound. Write it down. Next week you lost two pounds. Add it up. Write it down: "I just lost three pounds. Wow!" The following week you lost 1.5 pounds. Add it up. Write it down. Say it aloud: "Wow, I just lost four and a half pounds. Keep the momentum going. While at work you walk into the lunch room and see a ton of food. It's a pot luck. *Yikes! OK – think: Eat moderately.* Grab small napkin. Place small amounts of food on napkin. Hold napkin on your hand. Think of a regular size spoon. Limit your portions to this spoon. DO NOT stack your plate with a mountain of glob. Again, eat moderately. No one is telling you not to eat – I just want you to know what eating in moderation means.

Life is all about enjoying everything in moderation. Measure your calories every day. Learn to shop at the whole foods grocery stores. <u>Shift your diet to organic. Avoid foods with Gluten.</u> Avoid consuming processed sugar. Avoid eating some dried foods in boxes. Read about some genetically modified dairy products and their adverse affect on the human body. Eat healthy in order to have a healthy mind.

Along with a healthy mind, *eating the right chocolate will help your libido.* Chocolate contains the chemical Phenylethylamine. This chemical which is released in the pleasure center of our brains produces the same feeling that we experience when we are in love. It is recommended that you take *Phenylethylamine* as a supplement rather than eating a bunch of chocolate.

Find your nearest Whole Foods grocery store. If you live in the United States, Sprouts, Trader Joe's, and other food providers will give you a new perspective on what healthy food choices exist in this world. *It is never too late to begin eating healthy.* If you live outside of the United States or in an area where the previously mentioned stores do not exist, learn to plant a vegetable garden. There is no replacement to eating organic foods.

Chapter 3: Meditation and the Yoga Power of Rehearsal

You have to *learn to change your perspective in life.* If all that you
have been doing is working out great, then there is no need to
change. However, if your life is not going the way you want it to,
or if you want more out of life than what you have been getting,
it is time to set the Yoga Power of Rehearsal into effect.

What exactly is it? How can I do it? Will it affect all aspects of my
life? Many of these questions will be answered in this chapter.
The important thing is for you *to allow your mind to remain open
and flexible to this change.* I will teach you some unique ways to
train your mind and body and this new internal strength will
propel you to new levels of lasting happiness.

It is not enough to want. You must put action into any activity for
it to work. We, as human beings can think about things all day
long, however, unless we put coordination, balance, and action
into practice, our lives will not change.

*Resilience and constant personal strength - not large muscles will
get you through obstacles in your life.* The turtle will win the race
with constant and steady effort instead of uncoordinated
predictable bursts of momentum. Think about this for a moment.
One cannot build a high-rise building from the top. No – a strong
foundation must be formed that will support that tall building.
Work on your foundation! Begin to understand the powerful yoga

movement and how rehearsing such a movement will propel you into new heights. Build a strong foundation in your new life.

An advanced violin player did not become that way over night. No, he or she committed thousands of hours to that effort. Microsoft's Bill Gates and Apple's Steve Jobs did not become computer geniuses by chance. Gates and Jobs worked on their dreams by committing thousands of hours of working with computers.

Actors rehearse their plays or roles in movies. What about you? *Have you been rehearsing your new intended positive role in life?* How much time have you committed to this new role? How strong can you be? How strong will you be? We all have a surprising amount of inner strength that oftentimes only comes out when we want to do the things we seek to do.

A surfer wakes up early in the morning to catch the best waves. *The early bird gets the worm.* Most of us are willing to get up early to take that flight that will take us to our Caribbean vacation. But, what about short-term daily goals? How much personal effort will you put into these? Are you eager to become happier? **Know this:** *Positive change is possible only for those who want to change.* Small efforts or changes will add up to big changes in one's life. A drug user can kick the habit if he/she is willing to do so. A prescription user can lower and even discontinue use of a drug if they truly work on themselves. Learn to become eager to be happier in your life.

Have you put yourself first ahead of others? Can you learn to be selfish on those actions that will propel you to new positive heights? What is keeping you back? How long do you plan on staying back? Action includes the blinking of an eye. How many blinks do you do everyday? So – you say these are natural responses. The blinks keep our eyes moist and healthy. Yet, there are many other blink movements that you are ignoring in your life.

Are you eating healthy? Are you exercising? Are you purposely removing or distancing yourself from a toxic relationship? Are you breathing correctly? Are you working too many hours? Are you watching too much TV and negative news?

Are You Helping Others?

When I was a young boy my uncle asked me: "If someday you won the lottery, what would you do with that money?" I replied that I would pay off my parent's mortgage and put some money in the bank so they could live a comfortable life. When I became an adult my college professor asked me the same question and I gave her the same answer. Later in life I had a great job with a steady high salary. I visited my mom and found that her washing machine had stopped working and she had no money to fix it. Without being asked, I drove to an appliance store and purchased her a new front load washer and matching dryer. Years later I lost my job and my mother was there for me with daily meals and emotional support. She reminded me of the times I was there for her. *So, I ask you:* Are you in a position to help another person? What is holding you back? There is no time like the present to help those in need.

What about if you are rich? How much is too much? How much will you accumulate before you realize that material objects cannot bring you lasting happiness? Driving a nice car feels great, but then you're afraid to park it in most public parking lots. So – you Valet instead. You then tip the attendant and are on your way home. Is this the life that fulfills you? Instead of living such an empty life, drive your city streets and find a homeless family. Buy them a warm meal and watch their faces light up when you hand the freshly cooked food over to them. Random acts of kindness provides us natural levels of happiness.

Thanksgiving holiday should be more than once a year. Feed the poor and watch your self-esteem improve. Help the poor or those less fortunate than you and watch your happiness level increase. Do unplanned kindness events and feel the positive effects that each of these will bring into your life. *Don't wait until you are poor to want to help the poor.* Today is what you have. What keeps you from donating your old stuff to local poor families? How much stuff is too much stuff? Only you can answer those questions.

The Poor Person's Camp

I have been contemplating the notion that every person should enter a poor person's camp. The participant in this camp would voluntarily enroll and be partnered up with a homeless person for three to five days. No cell phones, no computers, no money, no contact with any of their family, friends, or personal contacts. No – the participant would learn how to live without the normal everyday benefits of their lives.

As they wake up, they would be hungry and thirsty. But, where to get some fresh water and some food? You couldn't buy food because you had to beg for it. An alternative would be to sift through restaurants' garbage bins in hopes of gathering others' leftovers. When one is hungry, even a bit of food out of a trash can tastes like caviar.

While in the poor person's boot camp, where would you hang out? Your clothes smell and most people do not want you near them. You could find a city park to lay down on a bench. How long would you lay on that bench before your stomach cramps reminded you that lunch was around the corner and you hadn't collected any food?

The sun will soon be setting and the temperature will drop to freezing. How will you keep warm? Where will you sleep? Will it be safe? Can you find others that can help you get through this one day. Yes, this one and very long day. You are on survival mode. You are on envious mode. You see others walking around wearing nice and clean clothes. They carry food in their hands.

The aroma of this food causes your saliva glands to begin watering. Yet, you have no food of your own to put into your body. No money, no one to call. Hopelessness begins to settle in. You are angry. How could this have happened to me? Why is this happening to me? *Why now?*

Do all or any of these questions sound familiar to you? They sound very much the same questions you asked yourself when you were employed and had money in your pocket. But, now – you are poor and broke. Pause. You have just learned a very important lesson. *Everything is relative in life.* The rich person has many of the same questions in their mind as does a poor person. A rich person worries about losing it all. A poor homeless person worries about this day being their last day on earth. A rich person stresses out about an investment that did not produce as much profit as anticipated. A poor person worries about how long they can lay down at a public park before the police or other homeless persons come to harass them.

Our lives are half chanced. One minute you are on top and the next minute you have lost everything and are living on the street.

The poor person's camp experience would teach many of you lessons that no advice or counseling would or could. You do have more than you realize. Wake up to your new happiness reality today.

How Happy do You Feel Right Now?

The answer to this question is the beginning you need to start your Yoga Power of Rehearsal transformation. A plant begins with a seed and such seed is watered and takes root. What size of roots you develop will depend on the size of your issue and amount of action and effort that you put into overcoming it.

You need to be aware that our happiness levels fluctuate with time. Still - even with this reality in mind, you must believe that you have the ability to turn your happiness level to high at anytime of your choosing. Yet, the interesting part of this concept is that there are no knobs to turn, no buttons to push, and actually these don't even exist. Yes, I am telling you that *happiness is the outcome of what you feed your mind and body.* Happiness cannot simply be adjusted by a button or turn knob. No; happiness is the result of what your mind and body is exposed to on a daily, weekly, monthly and yearly basis.

Today's News = Stress, Sadness, Anger, Frustration, Anxiety and Depression

You like to watch the news – but the news is full of negative material. This person died. This person was murdered. There were several automobile accidents. There are no jobs. This person was arrested for drugs and other crimes. So and so lost her job. I could go on this topic for days but the *reality is that daily news brings fear and negative thoughts into your mind.* How long do you plan to watch the news? How long before you realize that your mind and body is being exposed to the worst of the worst? Be it half an hour, one hour, ten minutes, or five minutes. *It doesn't matter how long you are exposed to this virus.* And yes, it is a virus; a virus that infects your mind and soul. This virus causes sadness, paranoia, depression, fear, hatred, anger, bias, prejudice, and artificial judgments. The only result that can come from watching the news is negative. You may try to say that you want to stay informed and that is a good explanation. However, if you don't realize that the daily news causes you negative outcomes, then you are in denial.

Being in denial is a very bad place to be. Being in denial blocks your ability to change your outcomes. Before you can begin the Yoga Power of Rehearsal, you need to wake up to the realities of the world. Not what your parents told you. Not what church or religion told you. No – wake up to see the reality of life. The phrase: "Garbage in, garbage out" is alive and well in today's society. Believe it and change it to fit your personal needs. Change it to *"Positive in, Positive Out."*

Let's move to cop shows. Really? This is how you spend your life? Watching crime and arrests, and jail, and people being murdered, stabbed, lied to, punched, robbed, raped, and violated? Yet, you say this is what you like? Think again. You may like this because it is stimulating certain feelings within you that usually do not get awakened. But, these are artificial and negative experiences. Yes – Negative. *Nothing positive can come from these TV shows.* You see people's lives being destroyed. They go to prison and get locked up for the rest of their lives. You get temporarily happy. Some get sent to death row. Others get released possibly due to lack of evidence or the fact that they were innocent. You may even get upset when someone gets found innocent in court. This feeling bothers you. You think that just because they were arrested, they are guilty. Wow! How much has your mind been tainted by all of this artificial media negativity?

When will you decide to remove this garbage from your life? When will you begin breathing fresh air? When will you awaken to the wonderful gift of life? Ride a bike lately? Have you sat by the ocean and mediated lately? Exercised lately? Eaten healthy lately? No? Then, why? What are you waiting for? What events need to happen for you to begin to feel the positive vibrations of this gift of life that you have been given?

Remove the illusions that are clouding your judgment. You don't need to have a heart attack to begin exercising, meditating, or eating healthy.

You don't need to almost die to begin living.

Yoga Power of Rehearsal Five Steps

Living the Yoga Power of Rehearsal involves five key steps.

Step 1: Recognition.
Step 2: Plan your escape.
Step 3: Water the roots.
Step 4: Assess and re-assess your progress.
Step 5: Return to step one and repeat the steps.

In **Step 1** we recognize that there are certain amounts of garbage that is entering our minds and bodies without limitations. *Too much of anything is not good.* Recognize that if you are eating too much, you need to slow down, reduce or minimize your eating habits. If you are too stressed out, recognize what is causing that stress and how can you minimize or remove this stress from your life. If you are unhappy or depressed, what is causing this condition and how can it be minimized or eradicated? Ultimately it is up to you to recognize the very condition or conditions that need immediate change in your life.

In **Step 2** we plan our escape. *It is an escape because you will need to create some distance and time between who you are and who you will become.* A sense of immediate urgency needs to be accepted and implemented. If you are in a toxic relationship, distance and time need to be implemented so that you can arrive at a more positive place. *Run like you have never ran before.* Push yourself not to return to the place that caused you such misery. But, before you run, plan the escape. Where will you live? With whom will you live? Don't leave a toxic relationship to immediately enter into another toxic relationship. No; plan your escape. A thorough plan will need to exist for you to withstand the course of time. In your escape plan you should include the free things and detours in life that can fill your time while you endure the change and pain that is and will take place within your body and mind. Some of these detours and free things are mentioned in this book.

Step 3 involves watering the roots. The roots I am referring to are the positive changes that you have implemented in your life. If you have stopped watching TV, tell others how this is improving your life. If you stopped an addiction, talk with other loved ones or a counselor how this change has improved your life. *Speak in positive language. You attract what you become.* Force yourself not to talk negative or complain about the issue or issues in your life. Know that most people do not like complainers. Instead, brag about your accomplishments and future goals.

Step 4 requires assessing and re-assessing what works in your life. We are in fact unique individuals and not all solutions work in all of us. What works for some people may in fact fail in others. As such, we must always be looking at any situation and understand what has worked for us and what has not. Keep what has worked and change or discard what has not. Don't spend too much time deciding on what to change.

If it is a positive change, your body will welcome it.

There are many stories out there that tell us that our bodies know what is good and what is not good for us. *If you eat healthy, you will feel healthy and act healthy.* If you eat garbage, you will feel like garbage and act like garbage. Even your skin pores will emit the smell of garbage. I don't have to go into much detail to explain to all of you what this means. You know in your hearts that you may have been eating foods that are simply not what you should be feeding your body. Yet, you continue this practice trying to see how far you can go before the next heart attack, or stress attack, or panic attack, or anxiety attack, or sudden death. How overweight must you become before you begin that diet? There is no time like the present to change to who you will become.

In **Step 5** you return to step one and allow yourself to cycle through all of the steps. As you do this, you will find that this *Yoga Power of Rehearsal method is now generating deep roots and positive change is in the air.* Your mind feels clearer. Your body feels healthier. Your stress level is down and you begin to notice small things in life that you had been ignoring. Yes, you are living in a very large world. This world is full of wonderful and mind cheering items. You begin to examine small flowers. Waterfalls sound louder for some reason. Healthy food tastes better. You look at the sky and notice the cloud formations and see the steady and unpredictable flow of shapes caused by winds and the earth's natural movement. You read and find that there are rivers near your home where you can go to read a book, fish, or just hang out and listen to the water sounds. Maybe you will drive a new road and find a new beach. The ocean is so blue. There are kids playing at the beach and their carefree personalities surprise you. One of them looks like you. Do you remember how fun it was to build a sand castle with your parents or siblings when you were young? Have you built a sand castle lately?

So, yes – Life is Half-Chanced. *The Yoga Power of Rehearsal seeks to transform you.* It seeks to awaken your inner soul. It seeks to teach you how to meditate and find quiet time to yourself where you can clear your mind and feel at peace. Once you arrive at this place, happiness is all around you. Others will see a transformation in you possibly before you do. Yes, internally – you will feel transformed but it will feel natural. *No drugs, no alcohol, no artificial potions. No! All the tools it takes to transform yourself already exist within you.*

Life is a Gift

Life is a Gift. Life is worth more than any amount of money on earth. You are already rich. So, what will you do with your gift? Will you seek out that which compliments you? Will you recognize that you are the captain in charge of your gift? Your hand is on the gearshift. You have the power at anytime to engage it to move forward in your life. It may take you a bit to find the clutch or have to put your foot on the gas pedal, but the reality is that once you make the decision to move forward in your life, a new adventure will begin. Such an adventure will show you that you are already living the dream. Where that dream takes you is totally up to you.

If there is conflict in your life, confront it. Those who have achieved happiness in their Yoga Rehearsal places know that life is a constant battle and you have to *be prepared to fight for it.* **Know this:** Nothing lasts forever applies to both good and bad events in one's life.   Life is a battle for anyone and everyone. The sooner you accept this very basic concept, the sooner you will be on your way to a positive transformation you never thought was possible.

Life is a game. This game includes many man-made rules as well as natural rules that many ignore along the way. Becoming happy and staying there is a natural rule. Each decision human beings make involves a certain amount of mystery, fear, and risk. We wonder if what we are trying to achieve will in fact turn out the way we want it to. *Risk, however, involves taking action.* Fear is part of the mystery that will keep you in the same place you have been up to now. *Learn to accept fear as it is also part of becoming adventurous and revitalized.* Take that public speaking speech class at the local college. Overcome your fear of public speaking and see how others can learn to overcome their fears. Only through experiencing risk and fear will you grow in Life.

Do You Live by the Beach?

The person who owns a house four blocks to the beach may at times forget that the beach exists. Really? What about the person who lives right on the beach? This person can see the beach everyday, yet – forgets or ignores the beach. Are you that person? Living four blocks from the beach is the same as living one or two hours from the beach. The choice to visit is always there for you to take. If you are alive, you have that choice. Drive or walk or ride your wheelchair to your beach!

"There are only two ways to live your life. One is though nothing is a miracle. The other is as though everything is a miracle."

Albert Einstein

When opportunity arrives in your life, grab it and hold on to it. You met that significant other that you love. Hold on to that person. Treasure that person. Appreciate that person. When sadness enters into any part of your life or relationships, treat these as opportunities to become a better person. With opportunities come challenges and these are the milestones you need to overcome in order to become stronger and happier. Once happiness arrives in your life, treasure it, admire it, pamper it, and enjoy it. You deserve it.

Multiple Positive Actions Bring Us Happiness

Happiness is not a single action- but a stack of actions that if followed on a daily basis, will bring you what you are looking for. Find those actions that bring you happiness and write these down. These will create a road map that you should follow into your new magical place.

Be bold and eager in looking for happiness. Be selfish when looking for happiness. Happiness is contagious. Once you arrive in the right place, you will be happy. Others will see you happy. You are happy as you are following your soul's purpose.

Don't be afraid to change. *It has been said that insanity is doing the same thing constantly and expecting a different outcome.* Force yourself to change. Push yourself to strive to make today better than yesterday.

Sit back and let go. Let go of the worries. Let go of the pain. Surrender to a peaceful place in your life. Listen to what your body wants. Listen to what your body wants you to remove from your life. Happiness is the outcome of positive and holistic actions. Follow those actions and allow this new happiness to immerse into your heart and soul.

Pure Happiness is radiating. Pure happiness is stronger than any other distractions. This is so because all humans strive to be happy and live in a happiness state.

Happiness is what your heart yearns. When you were created, realize that you were programmed to be happy. Sadness is a sign that your body and mind are not in tune on what it was meant to follow. Find that which brought you out of tune. Find that which awaits you in your life. *The best things in life are free.* Air, love, faith, beach views, water, and life. Feel those positive places that vibrate deep in your heart and bring that feeling up to the top. You are in charge of your body. Use that power to seek and transform you into the happy person you and I know you can be.

Giving, Seeking, and Being

Give and receive happiness as part of your daily routine. *Your body needs happiness like it needs food.* Practice searching for happiness on a daily basis. Teach yourself to seek happiness at least three times per day. The number of times will increase as you realize that being happy makes you healthier. Being happy makes you feel free. *Being happy makes you become aware of what you do have in your life.* You do have abundance in your life but you must allow it to surface in your life. Just because you don't see the submarine, it doesn't mean that it is not there. Once the submarine surfaces, you realize just how huge, powerful, and present it is. Happiness - like the submarine- can disappear at times. Stay focused. Bring your happiness submarine to the surface and show it off to the world.

When happiness disappears, send out daily notices that you want it back. *Let the world know that you seek happiness.* Let the world know you deserve happiness. Let the world know that happiness will arrive soon. Close your eyes and envision how happy you will be once happiness arrives. Ignore the distractions. Be in that place where that submarine will be allowed to surface. You have to be ready for change.

Stop being a victim. Abandon the fears. Abandon regrets. Abandon the anchors of yesterday. Abandon negative talk. Ignore your biases. Let go of hatred. Instead, find your passions. *If you want to change, you must first change yourself.* Love yourself first and trust that once you do this, you are ready to be loved by others.

It has been said that you shouldn't argue with the ignorant because they will knock you down and beat you with their experience. Identify those who are ignorant in your life and slowly detach yourself from those negative influences.

Always be present in who you want to become. Observe life with happiness in mind. Grow with your happiness in mind. Change yourself with happiness in mind. Your life becomes that which you seek. Attract that which provides abundance in your life.

Dream

Look at this dream you are living. We call this dream Life. When you look inside your dream do you see happiness? Is your heart yearning to be happy? What is it that is stopping you from achieving the best possible dream? The answers for these questions are already inside of your mind. Find that which fulfills you. *Push away and remove all that continually makes you unhappy in your life.* Move forward through time and space as a happy human being. Being happy feels natural. Act natural and you will begin to achieve that which you never thought was possible.

Chapter 4: Positive and Toxic Relationships

All human beings want to be seen and validated. As such, you should always expect good treatment from those you love. If this is not the case, do you tell those loved ones: "I love it when you walk all over me" or, "Thank you for always putting me down"? No; the reality is that you may think those words but most probably don't verbalize it to others. You must expect the best from those who love you. If this is not happening, then these could be toxic relationships. **Listen to me:** Avoid toxic relationships! You can try to fix these, but once you have determined that these cannot be fixed, then it is time to discard such negative energy from your life.

Some of you may believe, mainly due to early religious beliefs that marriage is forever. Well, I too believed that principle at one time. However, now, I believe that marriage is forever as long as the other person respects you, appreciates you, compliments you, supports you, encourages you, praises you, helps you, brags about you to others, forgives, and loves you. When I say "loves you" I don't mean that they say "I love you too" when you tell them: "I love you." No, you know what true love is. You sense it. You welcome it, you look for it, you anticipate it, and you deserve it.   Only use those words when you truly love a person.

Do not tell someone you love them unless you mean it. Those three words: 'I love you' must have a highly significant meaning in your life if you intend to validate what your loved one is telling you by using such a statement. What about when you begin dating? Date that person but only tell them you love them when you actually do. Don't simply rush to force something that isn't there. When you truly love someone, the words will come out of your mouth naturally.

Love must reverberate in both hearts for it to be real love. If one person is in love, but the other is not, then conflict is bound to exist. While I realize that some fall out of love and back into love… once a person in a relationship realizes that they have so much love to offer but the other person is not acknowledging, appreciating, caring, or loving them, then it is time to question, ponder, seek explanations, and ultimately make decisions that involve moving past these life hurdles.

The right relationship compliments us. The toxic relationship kills us. Positive energy is good. Negative energy is devastating. Can relationships be fixed? Yes. Can all relationships be fixed? No. **Know this:** *There are no accidental encounters.* Relationships begin in the positive energy field of who you are as an individual. As such, all relationship encounters aim to seek out that which is embedded within you. Once you find the place that allows your love to grow, you know that you are right within this intended purpose. The right relationship allows you to express yourself, allows you to grow, and provides you the same amount of love that you are giving the other person.

Real love is rare but not impossible to find. Once you find the right person, hold onto that person as they… like you, will endure changes along the path of life. Your heart knows when the real feeling of love is right. Love can be shared but should not be ignored. Similar to a plant, it must be watered and pampered or it will die.

Unconditional love is possible but rare. A new parent who looks into the eyes of a newborn baby will tell you that this child offers unconditional love. But, this is in fact not correct. That child loves a parent but it also has needs. As Abraham Maslow demonstrated in his Hierarchy of Needs Theory, all of us have personal needs. The baby will need food, clothing and, shelter. Without these, her love for the parent will deteriorate. This is similar to what happens when we ignore personal relationships and hope that they will survive the course.

Sadly, in some relationships when a person tells the other that they have needs, the other half may not be very loving. *"What? You have needs?* I had no idea of these needs when we met. How long will you have these needs?" Sound familiar? Instead of this attitude, we must accept that when there are challenges and needs in all relationships, we need to adopt the attitude of: "Let's grow together" to meet and work through those challenges and needs.

"Love has no meaning if it isn't shared"
Mother Theresa

What are you doing with your life? Once you have committed to being positive and happy, you will find greater passion and love that you never thought was possible.

Belief Systems

Our belief systems passed upon us from our parents and upbringing do not always provide us with the necessary power to overcome obstacles that unconditional love brings to the table. Real love is providing unconditional love to others but also accepting that there may be accommodations attached to this condition. Our mind at times pauses to question the validity or toxicity of our relationships. This is normal. Listen to what your body and mind wants or craves.

As human beings, we at times act like children when we don't get what we want. We at times compare our relationships to other relationships and wonder why we can't have this or that. Instead of doing this, you should be looking at your relationship to see if it can be fixed or if you should make a decision to move past this toxic relationship. You deserve better.

Being in a relationship is not always about the destination. No; being in a relationship may at times be the ongoing daily positive feeling that keeps you in it. Yes, there will be bumps along the road, however, if those bumps sum up to 50% or more of the time, then it is decision-making time.

It is possible to be happy in a relationship. This place exists in your person, in your heart and soul. When problems exist in a relationship, rather than jump to conclusions, ask yourself: "What is disturbing me?" The answer to this question is oftentimes your solution. Rather than try to fix the other half of your relationship, find that which bothers you. Find that which is damaging your positive energy and spirit. Find what can fix you.

Try not to fit the mold and please others. No, instead…you should demonstrate your uniqueness. This behavior will allow you to demonstrate your *Yoga Power of internal purpose.* So many people search for their purpose and ultimately many find that such purpose is already built into our beings. *I believe that we did come to this world with instructions.* Such instructions are built into our feelings. That which makes us happy agrees with those instructions. That which makes us sad, unhappy, unfulfilled, offended, depressed, disappointed, or hurt, goes against those instructions.

A smile is produced when we are happy. A frown presents itself when sadness arrives. Relationship mood levels often sway the pendulum between happy and sad. I say that if relationships were on a scale of 1 to ten when 1 is excellent and 10 is extremely low, where do you place on that scale?

At stage one you are happy, content, in a fulfilling and loving relationship. You may have casual arguments or minor disagreements that lower this feeling into stage 2 or 3 depending on the severity of the circumstances. A newly discovered affair may take you into stage 5, however, rocketing into stage 10 is extreme. Sure – go to stage ten if you wake up to find a burglar inside your home, however, you should never allow a loved one to rocket into level 10 for everyday relationship issues. *Anger and violence are simply not acceptable in healthy relationships.*

It is normal to visit areas 2 and 3 during normal arguments or disagreements. However, screaming at you, belittling you, yelling at you, and demonstrating anger towards you are not acceptable practices in loving relationships. Don't allow yourself to become a punching bag.

Location as a Condition of Happiness

Have you ever met someone who told you that in order to be happy they would need to fly to Hawaii? Are you that person? Do you try to convince yourself that the only way to have a vacation is to spend lots of money and take several planes in order to arrive at your destination? Maybe you have already flown to your favorite location only to find that what was waiting for you there was not much different than what you already had near your home or city.

Years ago I spoke with a couple who used to love getting away to Hawaii. They would take a plane and five hours later they arrived in beautiful Hawaii. The weather was mostly perfect each time they visited and both often wished they could visit more often. Then, one day a job opportunity moved the couple to San Diego, California. There they found endless beaches, walking trails, bike paths, stable weather, countless sights to visit, and new friends.   After living in San Diego for six months the couple scheduled and left to Hawaii for their much-anticipated yearly vacation. When they returned, each told me how Hawaii was not as exciting after they moved to San Diego, California. What they did notice was that the Hawaii food prices were much higher than those you could find in San Diego, California. Their out of state food selection was limited as Hawaii did not have as many diverse restaurants. Ultimately, I was asked why this happened.

As we grow up, we are told that if we do this or that, then we will be happy. If you live in the mid-west, a visit to Hawaii is all that you need to feel stress free. You are told this so many times that when you finally arrive in Hawaii your body responds by satisfying the very wish that has been embedded into your mind. A similar experience will happen if each time you are sick your parents tell you that you need to go to the doctor. Consequently, as soon as you arrive at the doctor's office, you immediately feel better. Your headache, stuffy nose, or other condition magically disappeared.

What I just described above is how the human body reacts to thoughts and beliefs that have been embedded into one's mind. We are told that the only place to become happy is Hawaii. Then, we must have Hawaii or we won't be happy. Unfortunately, this couldn't be farther from the truth. Your Hawaii or similar magical places already exist in your mind. **Listen to me:** No matter what city you live in, there are places to visit, things to do, and other activities to participate that will make you happy. *Location should never limit your happiness.* A prisoner who spent years in prison will miss his friends when he finally gets released. A prisoner can in fact be happy while incarcerated. If you believe that this can be true, you can free yourself from the thoughts, beliefs, fears, or statements that others have planted into your brain over the years that may limit your level of happiness.

Celebration Garden

So, where is your celebration garden? Where is that place that makes you feel complete? Have you found it yet? Have you found it before but now are unable to return? Know this: Whether you found it before or parts of such a place, it still exists within you. You can close your eyes and be there right now. No plane or train tickets needed. No money needed. *You can close your eyes and meditate and visit that very place now.* As you close your eyes and arrive there, do you realize that it is as beautiful as it ever was? Now you actually appreciate that place even more. Life has thrown you some obstacles and such obstacles now prove to you that this special place continues to offer the healing, peacefulness, freedom, joy and love that you know has always existed within you.

Gratitude and Inspiration

You have to be your best cheerleader. Consequently, you must learn gratitude and what it means to be inspired so that you will endure the natural course of life. Celebrate all wins, all achievements and, be grateful for what this life has provided you. Can you breathe? You are breathing free air. Can you see? You have the gift of sight. Are you blind? You have the gift of imagination. Can you think? You have the gift of free thought.

All of the previously mentioned qualities are presented intentionally as a way to inspire you. *Do not focus on what you don't have.* Instead, inspire yourself by focusing your thoughts, talents, and actions on what you do have. You have possibilities and these should always be converted into opportunities. Inspiration can come from others but it is best when it comes from within you. *Don't wait for others to inspire you.* No; you must learn to inspire yourself every moment of every day.

"You can't wait for inspiration. You have to go after it with a club."

Jack London

So, your boss yelled at you. Inspire yourself by being grateful that you have a job. Update your resume and begin looking for other jobs. The choice is always yours to make.

So, you ate fast and unhealthy food knowing that you were on a diet and are feeling down. Inspire yourself to become a better person and drive past this fast food place the next time you drive down this street. As you drive down that street, find a healthier place to buy food or eat at. The choice is always there but you must be ready to move on it. Action is required for change.

Demonstrate gratitude for all that has been provided for you in this life. Stare at a mirror. Say your name out loud. Then, add these words: "I know that I may not say this enough but you are a unique individual. Others like you. This life has given you both challenges and opportunities but you choose to stay on the positive so that those opportunities will turn into accomplishments." Life is what you make of it and by being persistent at staying positive; you will attract what you become.

Gratitude Meditation

Learn and practice daily meditation. Find a quiet place that you feel comfortable in. Sit on the floor and if possible cross your legs. Place the palm of your right hand on or near the right knee and the palm of your left hand on top of your left knee. Relax. Take slow and deep breaths. As you exhale close your eyes slowly. Each breath relaxes you more than the previous.

Your goal is to reach that magical place that only you know exists for that very moment as you meditate. Find the most comfortable position that will allow you to enter this meditative state. As you reach your high moment of relaxation, allow your eyes to stay closed as you begin to focus on your breathing. Slow and personal inhaling and exhaling brings with it good feelings. *Allow yourself to slip onto that private place which only you have found.* Continue to breathe slow deep breaths knowing and believing that such breaths bring positive feelings to you and actually pushes away negativity.

Each time a negative thought enters your mind, learn and discipline yourself to fade it away or re-route it to the trash bin. This is not the time to deal with any negative thoughts. No; this is your time to perform your daily meditation. Such meditation should be about replenishing your positive supply of happiness and bringing you relaxation and fulfillment. *Today is a new day.* Yesterday has passed and you choose not to dwell on it. Tomorrow is an exciting possibility. As you exhale, push out any frustrations or insecurities that you may be feeling.

Steady relaxed breathing takes practice. Just like exercise, you may only be able to begin with five minutes of meditation each day and then increase that time as your mind and body get used to this state. As you continue to breathe, allow yourself to think of the opportunities that await you. You can see smiles on your loved one's faces as they see you approach. They are happy to see you and give you lots of hugs and praise. Everyone is happy that you have arrived. You are loved. *You are cherished and appreciated.* Now, you move past this warm crowd and you are back at that peaceful place you have chosen at the start of your meditation. Listening to your breathing calms you. This breathing comforts you by taking you to deeper fulfilling and nurturing places. As you approach these places during your meditation, learn to value and allow them to consume your well-being. Learn to numb out the pain and to allow positive feelings to travel throughout your entire body.

Join a Yoga program that fits your lifestyle.

Learn to block out distractions. Daily gratitude meditation is an activity, which allows you to enter into a relaxed state that may be foreign at first. However, with time you will see that this practice will allow you to become a magnet for those things that you want to attract. *This is your moment. Cherish it.* Work on it. Seek out the best meditation pose that relaxes you. Discipline yourself to do this everyday. You may have to wake up 30 minutes early to do this. **Do it.** You may have to do it while the kids are still in bed. **Do it.** You may have to meditate in your parked car during your work lunch hour. **Do it.** Do what it takes to travel to a place that will heal and improve your mind's positive spirit each and every day. Your car needs gas. Daily meditation is your body's fuel that is designed to propel you to new heights.

"Clouds come floating into my life, no longer to carry rain or usher storm but to add color to my sunset sky."
Rabindranath Tagore

Daily gratitude meditation allows you to deal with daily circumstances, which require decisions while at the same time repel or push away people and circumstances that mistreat you or fail the see the true potential happiness within you.

Every single person on this earth is dealing with circumstances that may be affecting their well-being on a daily basis. You are not alone in this plight. No, without knowing it personally, you and others are all enduring circumstances that seek out answers to everyday problems or issues. Life is in fact about working through these issues and daily meditation gratitude sessions will provide you many of those answers. Whether you choose to do five minutes every other day or once a week, you will ultimately see a difference in the way you think, act, and treat others.

Chapter 5: The Prescription Pill Roller Coaster Ride

Roller coasters are fun. But what if you could never get off the roller coaster? Instead of a three-minute thrill ride, the roller coaster experience continued for hours, days, months, and years. At which point would you make the decision to get off that ride?

Most prescription pills are poison for your body. Would you intentionally put poison into your body? Many of you are doing so everyday. You are making the drug companies rich. You are putting your body on auto-pilot. *You are ignoring life.* You are numb. You are ignoring your loved ones.

Your kids or friends see you as a mindless robot. You take pills to sleep. You take pills for anxiety. You take pills for depression. You take pills for headaches. You spend lots of time at the local drug stores looking for the best medicines to help you with sinus pressure, colds, allergies, back pain, etc. It is time to begin thinking healthy and learning about natural medicine. Have you eaten an apple lately?

Have a headache? Drink water. Getting too many colds, wash your hands and take your daily vitamins, eat healthy, and exercise. Get a good night's sleep. *Stop shaking people's hands so much.* Clean your computer's keyboard with a disinfectant if others share it with you.   Go on the Internet and look up Don Tolman. Listen to his lectures. Learn what foods your body needs to stay healthy. Avoid visiting doctors on a weekly basis.

Be careful not to allow your work life to consume your entire life. Live a balanced life. On your days off, stay away from your work site, computers, smartphones, and the Internet. Never volunteer to work on your days off. Go for a walk. Find a new trail near a park. Ride your bike. Feel the sun and wind on your face. Force yourself to smile. Go swimming. Play a sport. Join an affordable gym and schedule set times to work out. Take regular showers.

Doctors Practice Medicine

Medical doctors are human beings who studied and passed some tests to make them doctors. Yet, many of their diagnosis are guesses. Yes, simple guesses. They examine you, then they guess: Hmmm... should I prescribe them an anti-depressant, or an anti-biotic? Should I prescribe them anti-anxiety medication or increase their current medication level? *Doctors practice...yes - practice medicine.* Think about it. The honest doctors will tell you that most of the time they could just tell you to get some exercise, lose weight, drink more water, eat healthy, stop smoking, stop wasting your life in front of the TV, stop overeating, and stop working late or overtime hours. But, no – instead, they prescribe you unnecessary medications so that you will return to their offices a week or month later with side effects. Yes – side effects. Read the labels: "This medicine has been known to cause internal bleeding, dizziness, vomiting, diarrhea, and even death." So, the question is: Why are you taking this poison? There is a reason why they say that doctors are practicing. They are practicing on your body. The risks you take by taking some of these medications far outweigh the benefits of many of these man-made synthetic drugs and poisons.

My disclaimer to the previous advice is that I realize that there are some medications that must be administered to those who simply cannot live a normal life without taking control of their mental, physical, or psychological issues and needs. However, it is my personal opinion that you should consult several doctors before you choose to fully accept their final recommendations. Choose the recommendation that feels right for your body and mind.

Recently, I was asked to take a medical survey in order to get a free gift card. I was intrigued by the experience since the survey was aimed at collecting medical information and providing other current medical information for patients who are contemplating on getting any type of surgery. The survey began by asking: What type of surgery are you considering? Then, it gets into small short videos that aim at educating the patient on the fact that not all surgeries are mandatory and that there are choices...or alternatives to such surgeries. The videos and questions constantly bombarded the points that the doctors' choices or recommendations were not necessarily the best for all patients. *Interesting!* This survey was taken in early 2014. So, yes – I am here to tell you that you are the best person to provide healthy decisions for your own body.

Don't Take Life Too Seriously

Be yourself - Be positive - Be flexible – Be humble - Be unpredictable - Be grateful for the life that you have. Be patient, yet – *be persistent about your life's happiness goals.* Have you worked on them today? Yes. Good. No? Why not? Is what you are working on right now going to make you happier? If so... continue please. If not – STOP IT. Focus, focus, focus. Be responsible to your needs. We all have needs. Some more than others. Yet, you... as the captain of your ship, know what needs you have and have an idea on how you will achieve these needs.

As you work to achieve these needs, have fun – make yourself laugh. Find the things that make you laugh. It is okay to laugh at yourself! **Laughter is natural therapy**. Laughter is personal and contagious. If you walk around with a smile on your face, others will want to be like you. Others will wonder why you are so happy. Others may even ask you: Why are you so happy? You reply: Because I am alive. Each day is a gift. I'm enjoying my gift.

Bosses Set The Tone

One third of our lives are spent at work. If work is bringing you sadness, you need to realize just how sad you are becoming. But, this section is more for bosses that it is for regular employees. Bosses are at times the main source of many negative feelings at work. If you are a boss or supervisor, pay close attention to this section.

Are you a boss or supervisor? How exactly do you treat your employees? Are you a jerk? Are you a negative Nancy? Are you a micro-manager? Are you grumpy, obnoxious, depressive, offensive, or destructive in your actions and daily behavior? Do you utter mean words when dealing with your employees? Why are you like this? Do you realize what you are doing to others? Do you realize the permanent damage that you are inflicting on others? Why did you not approve your employee's vacation request? Why did you object to that new modified schedule that would give everyone a permanent three-day weekend? Why do you constantly shoot down others' ideas? Why is it that you always have to be right? Why do you micro-manage others?

Know this: If what I just described is you, you are in fact heading for disaster. Good people will be harmed by your negative attitude. Great employees will gradually abandon you or the company.   Your relationships with family and other close ones will become irreparable. Is this what you aspire to be? Who or what made you this way? Could you change your behavior? What would it take to change? Today seems like the day you could change.

As I mentioned earlier in this book, the *positive change has to begin with you.* Others can give you advice, direction or suggestions, however, you are the captain and the choice to change must originate within your being. Don't wait for a tragic event to become a better person. Learn to be kind to others. *Learn to be humble!* Become aware of what your employees are enduring in their lives and do something to make it better. A kind gesture goes a long way. You, as the boss or supervisor must be the change agent that makes being at work a pleasant experience.

If possible, allow some top performing employees to leave work early on Fridays. Create a file to keep track of employees who have gone above and beyond their call of duty. Complete commendation letters to those employees on a regular basis. Make copies of those letters for their personnel files. Help those close to you to become successful. Begin to work on long-term relationships. Plant the seeds you wish to reap.

If you were fired today, who can you call to your aid? Have you given some thought about this? If you became sick and had to admitted into the hospital, who would visit you there? Your position as a boss or supervisor is temporary. One day, some day, or today could or will be your last day at work. How will you be received if you return to your company after leaving your current job? When your employees run into you at the grocery store, how will they remember you? Did you congratulate your employee on the recent birth of a baby? The purchase of a new house? Recent marriage? New car? Or, have you provided support to those employees who have recently underwent a divorce, separation, cancer treatment, loss of a home, or news of impending illness?

As a boss, please know that you are not alone. You attract what you become. **Learn to become humble.** Stop micro-managing your employees! Learn to be a warm and compassionate person. Glue a natural smile on your face. Learn to relax a bit. Leave your office door open. Learn to keep secrets when asked by your employees. Do you understand what it means to keep your word? Keep your promises so that others respect your word and your presence. Grab and hold every opportunity to help others.

By recognizing others, you will become recognized. You will be appreciated, respected and admired. Today is a new day. It is time to become a new and improved person.

Chapter 6: Depression – A new Approach

Have you ever met someone in your life that constantly looks to understand their life's complexities? Not only do they seek to understand them, but they tend to over-do-it. They talk about it, complain about it, get upset about it, and they just won't let it go. These people seem to attract the most 'negativity' that life has to offer them. You give them advice, then the next day they are still talking about the same issue, plus - now they have two more complex issues that just surfaced. As they walk away from you, you feel drained. What just happened? Well, some people are inherently unhappy and nothing you can do or say will change that. But, what if you are that person?

We must live our lives in places where we can find peace and tranquility that eventually leads to steady happiness.

As a college professor, many students would walk into my office or email me with all types of personal problems. A group of these students would constantly discuss their ongoing personal battles with school, work, and personal life and often times blame their backgrounds, parents, family, or friends for their demise. I would always listen to these stories and offer various types of approaches on how to deal with various life issues.

But - Let's face it - Stop living in the past. Stop blaming others:

Parents, friends, and society for your own failures. Accept that life is about setting goals, accomplishing those goals, and either celebrating accomplishments or learning from your mistakes and failures.

You have the power to control and deflect depression. For those who are reading this and have suffered from it, you know what depression is...and you know when it is coming. So, when you feel that it is coming, do what you have to do in order to keep it away from your body and your emotional well-being.

Force yourself to think positive. Force yourself to laugh, watch funny YouTube videos or Vines. Avoid....yes – *Avoid other people who are depressed.* Depression is contagious and truly damaging to the human soul. Depression knows no boundaries as it affects the poor, the rich, and everyone in between.

Everyday we are presented with situations that we have no control over. The way you respond to these situations will shape the person you will eventually become.

Positive and persistent will Power is the Key! There is no such thing as: 'I did the best I can.' When fighting depression, you can always do better.

In law enforcement survival training, officers are taught to never give up. They know that in their line of work many will face challenging obstacles as well as threats to their lives. Many survive personal physical attacks, shootings, and other critical incidents that oftentimes puts their survival instincts to the test. These instincts often drive a wedge between what the actual threat level is versus what the level is perceived to be.

In suffering my own depression after losing a well-paid and

highly successful job, I experienced a feeling where my mind wanted to keep living but my body had given up. I later learned that this feeling was a product of a heavy level of depression.

Depression is an interesting topic. I have personally known several people in my lifetime who suffer from depression but simply refuse to accept that they are suffering from this very common condition. They feel that if they deny it, or pray about it, the condition will simply go away. Well you know what? No! The first step in fixing this deadly (yes, deadly) condition is to recognize it. Read about it. Understand it. Once you understand that you may be suffering from depression and have read about it, and understand it, you will be equipped with the right tools for the right moments.

Once you recognize the early signs that depression is comin' a knockin'..... you must act and act quickly. Now that I understand what depression is, I have trained my body to respond in ways to combat it. Don't let the roots take hold.

Laughter is therapy – Use it!

You, God and Free Will

I don't proclaim to have all of the answers for your life's problems. I know that some of you who will read this book will be going through some of the worst times in your life – just as I have experienced on a personal basis. But, – again, *who is in control of your body?* You and God are. But, get this: God gave us all free will. So, use it. You are in fact solely in control of your body.

As soon as you wake up, Get up! Get in the shower, sing in the shower, put on some workout or upbeat music on your music player. Do not listen to public radio. Do not turn on your TV. Eat healthy food! Eat organic fruit! Put on clean and relaxing clothes. Go get some fresh air. Go for a walk. Make small goals in your life. Go to new places aimed at exciting and stimulating your visual and other sensory inlets. Sit facing the sun for five to ten minutes each day and allow natural Vitamin D to penetrate your body.

Compile a list of all of the positive things in your life. The list may be short initially, but eventually, it will grow. Write down a friend that once helped you. Write down a boss who was caring and did a good deed for you or another person. Think of local places that you would like to visit. Research the welfare department and if you don't have a job, apply for free benefits. Eat well and regularly. Take natural / organic vitamins. Exercise and do it regularly. If possible, join a Yoga program in your area.

Focus on what is positive in life. Force yourself to stop thinking negative thoughts. Every time a negative thought comes into your mind, immediately replace it with a positive thought. Force that positive thought to stay at the top of your "thinking list of items." It will take work, but you can do it. Look into Hypnotherapy if you need help doing this. Here is a link that may help you get started. (www.hypnomatters.com)

If you're living in California, check into a program called WIC (Women, Infants, and Children Supplemental Nutrition Program). This program will help if you have children and they need milk, cereal, cheese, and fruits. Every little bit helps. Other states may have similar programs through their community social services departments. Don't hesitate to apply to a Welfare program in your state that will put food on your table. Ignore what others may say about going on welfare. The reality is that when you are on survival mode you must use all of your available resources to stay alive. *Use all of your available resources.* Live Life!

I told you earlier in this book not to watch TV. Well, some of you will say that you like to watch TV just before going to sleep or shortly after waking up in the morning. OK, let's do this: If you must watch TV, watch a funny show (Married with Children, Mister Ed the talking horse, That 70s Show, or a Discovery Channel wilderness show, a travel show, a documentary on new technology, a mechanics (how to) show, and for some of you (as it worked for me) the Home Shopping Channel. Although I did not buy any of their items because I was broke, I enjoyed the level of enthusiasm that they presented in all of their products. Each time a product came out, the speaker would make it seem like it was the best, most innovative, unique, complete, fail-safe, and appealing product on earth.

Set your timer on your TV so that it doesn't stay on all night. A good rule of thumb in terms of time to watch TV before going to bed is no more than one hour. In an ideal setting, your TV should not be in your bedroom. You can in fact train your body so that once you enter a bedroom without a TV, your body knows that it is time to go to sleep. Listen to calm meditation music before going to sleep.

"You never know how strong you are until strong is your only choice"

Bob Marley

Don't Believe Everything that You Think

If you work a normal dayshift schedule, do not eat any food past seven in the evening. The main reason for this is that your metabolism slows down at the end of the day and your body simply will not burn up those calories at the same rate while you are sleeping. Eating just before you go to sleep is a recipe for gaining weight. Learn that it is acceptable to stop eating a few hours before you go to sleep. You should keep a bottle of water close to your bed in case you get thirsty or feel like you must have something to drink before going to bed or during the night.

Avoid drinking alcohol as the chances of you turning into an alcoholic during the depression stages of your life is very high. If you must drink something that resembles alcohol, drink a chilled cup of apple cider during the day.

Lastly on my recommendation list is to avoid or minimize taking anti-depressants. I know that with so many of you taking these on a daily basis, you are saying: "What? Stop taking these pills? You are CRAZY!" Well, the reality fact is that these small pills have a way of 'numbing' your natural feelings. When you numb your feelings too much, you are also numbing others near and around you and eventually they will push you away as you will begin acting like a person without a brain.

Think about this: Have you ever heard someone say "He was so cold of a person...heck, he didn't even cry at his parent's funeral" or, "When his mother told him she was dying of cancer, he told her that he needed to get back to work as there were several urgent projects that needed to be completed by the end of the day." Yes, I know that as you read these sentences some of you are relating to what I am telling you.

So, will it be easy to get off anti-depressants? No. But, is it possible? Yes. Should everyone get off anti-depressants completely? No. Have I confused some of you at this point? Possibly. Always check with a tenured and highly respectable medical doctor to learn about the proper ways of getting off or reducing your anti-depression medication. It can be a roller coaster experience but at some point you need to wipe away the fog and begin to see life in a clear and sober manner.

Ok, let's put it all into a clear perspective. If your depression is so severe that you have to take anti-depressants as a way to allow yourself to survive without losing your mind or committing crimes, you should continue taking your medication as prescribed by your doctor. Some medical depression conditions require constant and daily medication and the following advice is not for these type of people with those specific conditions.

A middle aged professional working man once told me that his life at times got so stressful that each day began with the feeling of being on top of a snow mountain and then - on his skis - beginning to slide down that mountain and being unable to stop. The only stop came at the end of the day when he finally went to bed. After realizing that he was suffering from anxiety and depression, he did go to a doctor who prescribed him a low dose of an anti-depressant. This low dose prescription still allowed him to function while at the same time managing and decreasing his anxiety and depression levels. After some counseling and hypnotherapy, he was eventually able to completely get off his medication and take control of his life.

While I know that some people take anti-depressants for valid reasons to cure severe depression conditions, I also know and believe that many people simply take anti-depressant pills to numb their lives from the daily routine of common ups and downs.

Research Don Tolman. He will give you a new perspective on what prescription pills are doing to your body and mind.

Have you ever flown in a commercial airline? Or taken a Greyhound bus ride? Do you want the pilot and driver of those two vehicles to be alert at all times? Why? Probably because if the pilot or bus driver were not alert, accidents could and will happen. So, think about anti-depressants and what they do to the human body. These products numb our feelings and often times – our physical actions. I personally feel that many of these anti-depressants are the reasons so many people commit suicide every year. When your feelings have been numbed, jumping off of a bridge is no different than going to the grocery store to buy some groceries. You enter the store to buy food because you are hungry. The suicidal person jumps off the bridge because he or she is depressed and highly disappointed in their life and seek an end to the constant pain.

Some of you who may be more academically qualified to understand depression may be reading this and thinking: "How can you compare the two situations? After all, one is totally absurd and the other is very common and acceptable. Well, in my personal opinion, having gone through my own depression at the very worst time of my life, I found that anti-depressants numb our feelings so much at times....that the absurd becomes the acceptable. And how does this apply to you? Well, you have choices. You can continue to live your life in a blur, merely breathing air in and out and waiting for the day your body will shut down... or you can choose to make some changes and begin living life – the positive way it was meant to be lived.

As stated by Doctor Bruce Lipton in his research in the Power of Consciousness, living a positive life includes looking at anything and everything that is in harmony with your life and avoiding or pushing away anything that brings disharmony to your life.

Recipe on how to avoid Depression:

What not to do:

- Don't sleep in.
- Don't stay indoors too long after waking up.
- Don't watch the news.
- Don't read newspapers.
- Don't watch TV.
- Don't listen to public radio.
- Avoid hanging out with depressing individuals.
- Don't spend too much time alone.
- Don't hang out with others who are depressed.
- Don't think about suicide.
- Religion and a strong belief in God is important – However, don't use God as a crutch. Embrace your religious beliefs and attend church as often as you can or as often as you need to feel a connection with the all mighty. If you accept that he created you, then you know that he wouldn't want you to go hurt yourself in any way shape or form. He is always with you, regardless if you go to church regularly or hardly ever.

Don't be ignorant. Realize that evil exists and also lives within us. You must know that there are two pit bulls living inside your body. One is a good pit bull – the other, a bad pit bull. Once you realize these two – very different pit bulls or forces exist in your body, then you begin to realize how you can change your life. *It is your duty to protect the good pit bull from the bad pit bull.* Remember that failure to feed the good pit bull will make the bad pit pull stronger. As such, always feed the good pit pull.

Eat WELL

The phrase: *'Garbage in - garbage out'* is just that. You get out of your body what you put into it. You must eat regularly (breakfast, lunch, dinner) and eat well when you do eat. Plan your meals. Eat fruit. *Eat an apple a day.* Set your clock alarm to remind you of these meals. Our bodies need fuel. Our fuel is food. This sounds like a simple concept, yet - so many people don't realize the importance of this daily requirement.

If we don't feed our bodies, they tend to begin shutting down or displaying malfunctions. The malfunctions I am referring to are headaches, pains, colds, flue, and other diseases that the human body will experience due to having a low level immune system.

Don't Give Up Control

You are the captain of your own body. God gave you this body to do great things. Don't focus on the negative aspects of your body – instead, use your influence for the good of humanity. Even a person born without any arms or legs has a purpose in life. Find your purpose.

Exercise

Exercise will do for you what many prescribed medicines can't or won't. If you are like me and enjoy reading about cars, you will know that as you peruse the classified ads, you will see many cars with high mileage where the seller says: "Mostly highway mileage." This statement refers that the car wasn't doing much stop-and-go activities, but was in fact cruising at a steady speed for long distances - possibly to the owner's work place. Highway miles then - are not considered as rough on a car as miles driven mostly in town during stop and go traffic.

Most police cars have stop-and-go miles, plus those cars are parked for long periods of time with the engine running. The odometer says 90,000 miles, but the hour meter check shows that the vehicle's engine was left running/idling for at least 45,000 more miles. In terms of low mileage cars, you need to ask yourself if the car was parked for too long of periods. A car that sits and doesn't run - often will begin having more problems than a car that is driven regularly during the high number of highway miles.

Similar to these previous examples, our human bodies should not 'just sit' as the mere sitting does not generate the necessary nutrients that our body needs to survive. We need vitamin D (from the sun), we need our body to produce several natural ingredients such as Dopamine, Gaba (Gamma Aminobutyric Acid) and exposure to laughter which produces endorphins that makes us naturally happy.

When you exercise, you 'run' your body to higher levels than it's used to - thereby producing the needed ingredients to keep it healthy. I can't say enough about the importance of exercise. Start slow and take it easy. Consult a doctor if you have to - before you begin exercising. Drink plenty of water and take your daily-required vitamins. Get up from the couch and exercise. *One hour of exercise a day will in fact change your life.*

Once you realize that your life is not as depressing as you have led yourself to believe, *look for your personal passion in life.* What are your interests? What are you passionate about?

Have you found your passion yet? Don't hold out on this area or you will miss out on life. It may sound like a cliché, but life is meant to be lived with positive purpose. Those who hesitate to make positive changes in their lives will often pass up hidden opportunities and rewards.

Most people who have lived a full life also realize that the world is not always full of sunshine and colorful rainbows. No matter how successful you are, there will be days that you will find it difficult to go on. There will be days, such as are described in this book, that little energy will be left to go on. But you know what? You are in the pilot's seat of your own body. *You are the captain, who at any time has the power to switch on the engines and charter a new course in your own life.*

The weak will say: But, what about this? What about that? Well, "this or that" or the *"What IF" this or that will not make you a better person* – it will simply leave you on idle speed at the same location...while others, who have figured out how the transmission works- engage it to "Drive" and... fly past you in hyper speed.

You Become What You Think

People who believe in mediocrity will often times tell you to 'be realistic.' Well, if you understand this statement, then you must also understand the importance of ignoring people who offer that type of advice to you. *You need to ignore reality at times in order to achieve higher ground.* You become what you think. If you think at higher levels than what you are currently at, then you will achieve those higher levels with the right amount of effort and intended purpose. Fake it until you make it. *Aim High.*

I remember watching the documentary "The Secret" which was endorsed during an Oprah Winfrey show almost a decade ago. In it, successful people commented on how important it is to visualize where you want to be and truly believe that you can get there. A sample situation used during the testimonials was how when you enter a parking lot, if you want to find an open parking space close to the building, you must believe that there will be an open parking space close to the building. If you enter the parking lot thinking that there probably won't be any open spots near the building, then you probably won't find any. Consequently, if you think positive, then positive will follow you in your life.

It all boils down to the fact that you have to dedicate yourself to being better every day. Every day presents a new opportunity to excel and you need to have internal motivation for this to occur. Without constant personal motivation, life will beat you down to your knees and keep you there as long as you let it. You and you alone have the power to move past any situation.

Often times we are our own worst enemies. We focus on the damage instead of the opportunities. We allow society to determine how we will proceed forward instead of looking at all of the options and making a wise decision on which option to select as part of our future.

Winning in life comes with lots of bumpy roads and tempting frill exits. As you travel that road and life throws you some blows, do you realize what the blows are all about? These blows are tests. Tests of your will power and how you will respond to the challenges. These are tests to see who will be left standing once the dust settles. So, as these blows knock you down on your bottom, how long are you going to stay down? No – Get up. Get up and fight for a winner is not a loser and losers never win.

Often times we don't pick our battles – they pick us. As a fellow human being, I love you and want you to be successful. Don't be a coward and take the easy way out. Your decision will have a cancerous reproduction effect to people that you will leave behind. <u>So, fight, fight, fight, to not give up. Fight to stay the course.</u> Fight to make yourself happy and content for the Life that God has offered you. Accept what you cannot change. Regardless of what you have done… today – is a new day. Today is the day that you have the choice on how you will live the rest of your life. Take that choice. Don't look back. Your most important day just began.

From my email to my friend Mike:

I'm happy to hear that your life seems to be turning around and that you are finally putting some money in your pocket. Remember this: don't relax. Keep the same positive energy in you that allowed you to get back up on your feet, get your place, get a new job, buy your car and move forward. I have learned that when we ignore the things we cannot control and focus on what is available to us and that we have the opportunity to control... life becomes so much easier. Bryan

Henry Ford once said that *whether you believe you can or you believe you can't, you are right.* Hence, the power of anyone's perception is what precipitates change and whether that change will become positive or negative. If you repeat and ponder negative, you will be negative. If you ponder and think, and verbalize positive, you will become positive. You become what you practice.

Be or practice being eudaemonic. By doing so, you will produce happiness and attract well-being into your daily life. It isn't all about yesterday's party but the journey on how you arrived here. Today is your new journey – Treasure it!

Chapter 7: Positive Behavior takes work

Our daily behavior matters. Each day you turn on the Television you are immediately inundated by negative news. Bad news about murder, rape, mayhem, fires, natural disasters, crime, car accidents, domestic violence, theft, traffic delays, deceit, government blunders, and stock market declines. It is no wonder that the majority of people around you inherently have a negative perspective on life and gloom and doom look for the future. Sadly, many individuals begin their day watching the morning news as they get dressed for work. Before arriving at work they have been exposed to a number of sad stories. These stories include pain to those involved in the incidents as well as their families and friends. *Without realizing it, you absorb this pain into your body.* All of this happens before you get to work. You drive to work with sadness, and a subliminal negative weight on your mind that you simply don't recognize is draining your batteries.

It is time to recognize what the morning news does to your body. Once you recognize this, you can then change what your mind absorbs before you begin work. You can control the music you hear in the morning. You can control what your mind listens to in the morning. You have the power to change this behavior at your fingertips. Use this power to change to a more positive lifestyle. Such lifestyle will bring you newly found happiness.

You know what else? The music radio in your car does the same thing as the television set. *Paid commercials brainwash you into believing that life is full of doom and gloom and unless you do this or that, you simply will not make it through the week, month, or year.* The fact is that unless you recognize that behavior such as watching the television news and listening to your public car radio is shaping who you will become, you may never see a positive side of yourself that will provide health, tranquility, peace, satisfaction, optimism, certainty, adventure, love, opportunity, and happiness.

Our bodies are amazing works of art. We react, contract, and expand as a result of experiences that we present to and involve our bodies in. If we are happy, we produce more dopamine. Dopamine then spreads through our bodies like a natural drug that revitalizes and re-energizes the various parts of our nerves, muscles, and mind. So, how do you create dopamine for your body? Exercise seems to be at the top of the list. Start with walking and eventually work on various activities that allow your body to break into a sweat.

I recall going through a restaurant drive-through with my daughters. The line was long and the lady behind us seemed very stressed out with her own kids in their car. Lots of yelling was going on as the mother tried to settle down her kids. As I approached the pay window, I paid for her meal order. This is classified as a *random act of kindness.* Buying meals for homeless people, hungry children, and others who are less fortunate than us will bring you natural dosages of dopamine.

As mentioned earlier in this book, yoga and *meditation* also allows an amount of dopamine to be dispersed through our bodies. Subsequently, begin giving others *gratitude* each and every day. When you go to buy groceries, give the checker a verbal compliment on what he/she is wearing. At the bank teller window, compliment the employee on their smile, or their friendly personality, or how positive they were towards you. Make it a point to tell a person's supervisor how well they perform their jobs. At work, find a way to write some letters of commendation for your co-workers or support staff so that they are recognized for going above and beyond their call of duty. By praising others' positive behavior, you will create natural dopamine in your body, which in turn will cause you to feel positive about yourself.

It Is Easier to Smile Than to Cry

Praise others and you will make friends. I recall my oldest daughters in their early years in first and second grade. The teacher would have the classroom kids perform some classroom activities where the students had to work in teams and interact with other teams in order to process the various building materials. At the end of this activity, the teacher would have the students sit on the classroom floor in a circle and praise another student for what they observed to be positive behavior. Each student would tell others comments like: I like the way Brian treats me in class. He is always very polite. I like the way Emma helped me with gluing the project. It was hard work but she never complained. I like the way Hannah is funny. When some of us are sad, we can always count on her to bring us a smile. I like the way Maria tries to teach us Spanish. She will someday become a great teacher. I like the way Antonio helped each member on his team. He is always supportive and helpful. Without realizing it, all of these verbal offers of gratitude gave these young minds a natural dosage of dopamine. Each student realized that by praising others, they felt good about themselves.

A day in the year 2014

The year is 2014. It has been four years since I finished my long-awaited doctorate degree. Such an accomplishment came with too many sacrifices that I simply will not include in this book due to their negative tone. **Know this:** Anytime you are trying to accomplish such a heavy task in your life, it tends to consume each and every action. Your friends are affected, your family is affected, and yes – you are affected as you have chosen to give up some or… a lot of your free time to work on accomplishing: The Goal. This paragraph teaches you that time stands still for no one. Yes, getting my doctorate degree took four years out of my life, but you know what? That experience is now in the past. Four years in the past. We simply can't change the past. The only, underline only, thing we can change is the Now. Yesterday is too late and tomorrow is simply a possibility. So – learn to live in the now. Yes, have goals. Yes, have dreams. Yes, look towards the future. But, do not waste time thinking about the past. The road to being happy begins today. Today is the moment you have chosen to abandon the past and look forward to the future. Write this date down.

Consequently, abandoning the past takes work. Similar to learning a new language, being happy requires you to make some permanent changes in your life. Change the way you think and you will begin to see subtle differences. Change the way you act, the way you dress, the way you standup and others will begin to notice your positive changes. Now, remember, these changes are for you first. These changes must begin with your internal desire to change and eventually turn into actions towards that change. *Never say that you are changing for others as they too are going through their own changes.* You must become your own pillar. You must root that pillar deep into certainty and confidence if you are to remove the negativity from your being.

Doing nothing to change yourself will give you… zero results. Doing something, no matter how small or insignificant to others, will plant the seed that will reap the positive rewards. Hence, it is important to avoid having unrealistic expectations as these tend to distract you from what you want to accomplish in your life. *If what you have been doing thus far has not worked, then – change the way you think, act, and respond to life.*

On a side note, over the years of teaching college and university students I would have many of them approach me and tell me that they were depressed. The reasons for the depression would often include: family restrictions (lack of freedom), part-time or full-time jobs that were not a good fit, toxic relationships, lack of money, and boredom. Yes, they were bored with their lives, school, relationships, and life overall. What was my best advice to them? A question: Why are you here?

Why are you here? What do you want out of life? If you could change one thing in your life that would cost you nothing, what would it be? My advice is to follow my Yoga Power of Rehearsal list for the quickest changes in your life.

-Avoid watching TV.
-Avoid listening to the radio.
-Avoid being in toxic relationships.
-Find a job that you like – even if it pays you less money.
-Respect your family.
-Respect yourself first.
-Respect your true friends.
-Laugh and smile whenever possible.
-Don't take life too seriously.
-Don't live your life with the fear of what could happen.
-Listen to wise advise.
-Listen to audio lectures that promote a positive attitude. Do this often.
-Read books that encourage you to be happy and enjoy living life.

The previous list of advice assumes a few things: You must accept who you are and like who you are in order for your life to move forward in a positive manner. If you don't like where you live, what have you done to find another place to live? If you hate being home, have you visited some nearby parks? Are there any waterfalls in your city? Whether they are man-made or natural, the sounds and sights of waterfalls help you to relax. No waterfalls nearby? What about pet stores? Have you visited a pet store lately? Hold a kitty or small puppy in your lap. Play with them. Do you sense the innocence in their beings? Unconditional love, and production of natural dopamine for free.

Now, put the puppy or kitty back and go see the fish tanks. Look at a fish tank that has several fish in it. If you were one of these fish in that aquarium, how would you feel? The aquarium is small – plus, there are humans looking at you eight to ten hours a day. Here we have a huge ocean out there and this poor fish is limited to a small aquarium. Yet, can you see that he makes the best of it? He/she swims around looking at other fish, eating their daily meals, exploring some small man-made structures buried within the aquarium. So, now – think of how that fish would act if he/she were released into the ocean or a large lake? So much to do, so little time to do it. Right? Now, opportunities are abound. The small fish will surely take a while to adapt to this new large lake or ocean, but I'm sure it will do just fine.

It turns out that you are such a fish. You have limited your life to a small town, a small city, a small neighborhood, a small group of friends. You have forgotten that out there, all around us– there are opportunities waiting for you. Whether it is sinking your feet into a sandy beach, going for a walk, visiting a pet store, walking through a beautiful park near waterfalls or small ponds... **life is meant to be lived. Life is meant to be explored.** You need to begin your exploration. What is it you like that can be done right now for you? You are a Chameleon pillar. You can change yourself according to what is happening around you. You must begin the transformation process of changing from who you are to who you will become.

In reality, only a small percentage of what we do makes us happy. You know this first hand as, similar to days off, you only have a small percentage of time off from work. Well, it turns out that the silent part – what our brains think – plays a bigger part in how happy you will become. **Try this:** Find a quiet place in your life. (quiet park, bedroom, backyard, inside your car, etc.). Find a shady spot and sit down. Close your eyes. Imagine that you have just arrived in Hawaii. As you exit the plane, you take a taxicab to the beach. You walk out of the cab and immediately remove your shoes. You walk on the sand and feel the sand between your toes. There are sounds of small waves breaking nearby. An ocean breeze hits your face and you can hear the sounds of seagulls flying nearby. There are sounds of children playing as they throw beach balls back and forth to each other. The children run towards the water and scream as they feel the fresh ocean water. You can hear splash activity as the children use their hands to throw water on their friends. Then, all is quiet. The families have left and now you are left on the beach all alone. You look out towards the other end of the beach and see a couple holding hands as they walk on the beach near the ocean. This couple looks happy. Wait! You are one of the persons holding hands. You are happy. You have found your other half. There are no worries in your lives and this moment consumes your heart and soul. You feel wanted. You feel appreciated. You feel adored.

It turns out that the above story allows you to experience an important point I am trying to make. You don't have to leave for Hawaii to feel the experience of being in Hawaii. The warm thoughts and feelings, and sounds you heard and experienced are already in place in your mind. If you believe this to be true, you can make yourself happy now using the Yoga Power of Rehearsal method.

Meditate – close your eyes. You are at work and your boss has just told you that you are being promoted. The promotion means that you will double your salary but it only requires you to work one day at the job site. The rest of the week will be spent at the company's corporate center in Cancun, Mexico. The corporate center is actually a large beach house with a devoted staff that is there to pamper to all of your daily needs. The staff will cook daily meals, help you exercise in the large gym – overlooking the ocean. The new job includes a limo with a driver and a bodyguard. You will have several assistants assigned to your daily activities. Each of these assistants will help you achieve your work goals while supporting your every need.

Your optimism levels will often predict how you will arrive at such pleasant locations and internal feelings. Again, optimism takes work on your part. You have to ignore the negative and focus on the positive. Ignore the distractions! By visualizing the opportunities instead of the barriers, you will someday arrive at a healthier level of optimism that will benefit each and every action in your life. Happiness is possible if you let it happen.

Wellness, health, and safety

Wellness, health, and safety all play a key role in becoming a positive thinker. Search out activities that promote such healthy practices. Go on YouTube and listen to Don Tolman. He will guide you into a healthier living style. His advice to abandon prescription medicine will shock your conscience. He will tell you all about man-made medications and all the side-affects these are causing on a long-term basis on the majority of the population.

If you are a hypochondriac, you will have a tough time with Mr. Tolman's advice. He believes that side effects of synthetic medications are actually "effects." There is nothing about 'side' as they are actual 'direct' effects on your human body and mind. If you take prescription medication, which has these effects, you will eventually have to take other medications to counteract such short and long-term effects. Before you know it, your medicine cabinet will contain an array of medications that are actually doing more harm than good for your body.

Positive behavior as a direct link to happiness

Positive behavior also has a direct link to what type of relationships you are engaging in. If you are in a toxic relationship, you need to see if it can be fixed. If it can't be fixed, it's time to move on. Move forward with your life!

Have you ever been happy around a friend or family member and then someone walked up to you and began a conversation about doom and gloom? As they walked away, you felt drained and wondered: "What just happened?" Well, I have labeled these individuals 'energy-vampires.' There are many of these energy vampires in our society. Our bosses, our spouses, our kids, our significant others, and even some of our close friends all can be energy vampires. If you know of specific energy vampires in your life, you need to make a concentrated effort to avoid any exposure to them. You may believe that these individuals can be changed, however, the reality is that they are the ones who are in fact changing you.

You are meeting for coffee with an energy-vampire. Their cell phone rings and they answer it. You hear them say: "Well, I don't feel good, my back hurts, my body aches, I hate my job, I hate my life, my car is about to break down, and I dislike most of my friends." They get off the phone and you give them the look. They reply: "Oh, no- I didn't mean that I dislike you, I meant my other friends." So, next week, the same scenario takes place as you two are at the grocery store. You listen to the cell phone conversation as the same person tells the caller: "I feel like shit. My body hurts, my back is all messed up, no clothes fit me, my job sucks, my life is all messed up, my car broke down and I'm tired of getting calls from annoying friends who just don't seem to stop calling me." You listen to this cell phone conversation and begin to think that what I am telling you is true. If you hang around this person too long, you too will become just like them. You will talk like them, complain like them, and fail to act on your life – just like them. As human beings we often mirror what we see in our lives. If all we see is negative, then that becomes the norm and we become negative.

Friday Nights

This brings me to Friday nights. As many of you who read this book know, Friday evenings can either be positive or awkwardly negative experiences. Positive as another week just ended, or negative as you are sitting home all alone on Friday night wondering why nothing positive has happened today. Well, it turns out that similar to relationships and positive thinking, Friday nights take work. It takes planning, coordinating, and following up on who will meet you or join you or dance with you. You can't simply wait for Friday to arrive and do nothing – expecting that someone will ask you to join them for Happy Hour. You must reach out into the social circles early on to see what others want to do as a way to celebrate another ending to a long workweek. Talk to several groups and see what each is doing. *Have choices – make wise decisions, take action.* If you're tired of going out, stay home. If you're tired of staying home, coordinate with others so that you can go out, meet with people, and socialize.

While I believe Friday nights have strong significance in many professional people's lives, I will tell you that I have my strong beliefs on what "Happy Hour" is and what it is not. Most happy hours that I know take place at a bar, pub, or other social hangouts. These events often involve the consumption of alcohol and unhealthy food. Drunk people often have diarrhea of the mouth and this can at times affect relationships both at work and on a personal level. Alcohol affects people in weird ways and as an adult you should moderate this drug as it will have long-term effects on your life. To me, happy hour should be a time wherein you are having fun, enjoying yourself, and feeling self-fulfilled, naturally. If your happy hour includes too much drinking, too much risky behavior, then you should re-assess your actions and make the necessary adjustments to these life-changing events.

What about your job? We are told that if you work harder, you will be more successful. We are told that by being more successful, you will be happier. However, this couldn't be further from the truth. Accomplishments of success goals often require new and upgraded goal posts. Each time you accomplish one goal, your boss moves the goal post on you. If you were a mule, a stick could be tied to your head and a string hanging from the stick would hold a juicy carrot. You would walk endlessly towards getting closer to the carrot, but as you and I know – the space between your head and the carrot will not decrease with any amount of steps you take as the stick is attached to the same spot on your head. You are in fact walking on a treadmill. Life at times makes you feel like you are living on a treadmill. Wake up early, get the kids ready, go to work, work, pick up kids, come home, cook, go to sleep, wake up early, get the kids ready, go to work, work, pick up kids, come home.

I posit that you should not tie happiness and positive behavior with becoming successful. *You should be happy because you are.* You should be positive because you chose what information enters your brain and what information should stay out of your brain. Similar to the Hawaii examples that I discussed earlier in this chapter, your brain longs for happy experiences and oftentimes stresses out whenever you are going through negative experiences. In fact, stress is a real human killer in today's society. Stress is often caused by too many activities in too little amount of time. Deadlines, too much work, demanding boss or significant other, spoiled children, car problems, financial problems, etc. all tend to cause stress in our lives. Once you recognize what causes stress, you should begin a program to minimize or delete such activities from your life. We all recognize that it is not healthy to work seven days a week. Yet, some of you still do it. Have you not realized that your body needs at least one or preferably two days of rest each week? Have you not realized that unless you take some time to meditate and relax without tasks, you will burn out your body before it is ready to stop working? Have you not realized that stress can be managed and is highly curable?

If you minimize the amount of stress level in your life, you will find that your mind will think clearly. As an employee, your employer also knows that if you are not stressed, you will be more productive, healthy, and efficient. If your job requires "accuracy" as one of its duties, a decrease in stress will show an increase in accuracy. Yet, all of this can only be achieved if you work towards becoming a more positive person.

Chapter 8: Hypnotherapy and Meditation as a new storyline

Are you paying Attention?

Your teacher looks right at you in class and says: "Are you paying attention?
Has this ever happened to you? Maybe you heard your teacher asking other students that very question. Well, for now, I am your professor and I am asking you: "Are you paying attention?"

What is it that troubles you? What distractions exist in your life that is limiting what you can accomplish with your life? As a human being, are you able to take any piece of information in your life and determine what its significance is? Why is this information so important? How can this information benefit or hinder you? How can you transform this knowledge in some way so that it can someday make sense in light of all the other things that may be tumbling around in your mind?

Know this: You are in fact able to transform from a negative thinker into a positive thinker. You are able to stop watching TV and listening to the radio and instead – listen to what matters in your life. The advice I am giving you in this book is to be viewed as shortcuts to arrive at the end goal, which is happiness. The only way this advice and wisdom will work on you is if you believe in it and allow it to transform your mind.

Loneliness

How does it affect the human body? Similar to physical pain, it is real and you should know that this condition is actually temporary. You have the power at any time to join social groups that will help you find people that may have similar interests as you do.

Please note that when you were a child, being excluded from events involving your friends did cause a bit of discomfort. Yet, your parents, brothers, sisters, and friends, were there to help you get through it. However, when this happens in adulthood, the feeling can at times become overwhelming. Sadly, as an adult, you may not want to seek out help or understanding as to why you are not included in your immediate friends' social functions.

Take action to combat loneliness. Use the Internet to search for local social groups that meet on a weekly basis. Through such networking you will gain insight on the opportunities that exist within you local area. The closer you live to a large urban city, the more social groups you will find. Some groups are into sports, others into networking, entrepreneurship opportunities, community participation, or dating circles.   Each of these groups will open up doors into future possibilities. Explore such opportunities and you will see how your mind will change.

Do Not enjoy being sorry for yourself. Instead, take action! Find those opportunities that will allow you to contribute and be part of a social group. Look for your talents and see how these can help others. Through this process you will help others and they in turn – will help you. If you just meet one friend – this is important. If you meet more than one friend, it becomes of greater importance. Build on these relationships.

As I told you in prior sections of this book, force yourself not to feel or look down. *Do not re-hash your past. Live in the present.* Force a smile on your face. Take a shower and smell good for you and others to enjoy. Dress in clean and comfortable clothes. Brush your teeth, and gargle with mouthwash so that you will have fresh breath. These minor changes will allow others to be comfortable near and around you.

Take a shower everyday. Some of you don't want to wash your hair everyday. OK – I understand. But – your body needs to be washed everyday if you want to smell good for others. The human sweat and unclean odor emitted by your body is one of the first causes that will push others away from you. This includes loved ones. As such, you need to pay specific attention to this important detail. Enjoy a quick shower or a bath early in the day and allow your pores to breath and remain healthy.

Other minor details include getting a hair cut, a shave (if you're a man), or shaving your arms and legs if you're a woman. Clip your nails. Pluck those annoying hairs under your chin or on your face. Clean your nails as no one likes nails that have dirt under them. Use a Q-tip and clean the outside area of your ears. Are the clothes you are wearing in agreement with those around you? PERSONAL HYGIENE is a major factor in getting accepted by others in our society. Don't ignore these tips that I just gave you. Instead, find some great smelling soap, shampoo, conditioner, body wash, toothpaste, and mouthwash. Visit your local drug store to see what products are available for you. Take pride on how you look and others will notice you in a positive light.

Back to that smile. Glue a permanent smile on your face. Smile at the person on the check stand. Compliment them on how they look, how they were very helpful, how well they know the cash register, how great they look today, etc. *Make others happy and you will begin to feel this positive energy coming back to you.* We all like compliments especially when they come in surprise form. A person who is not expecting a compliment will feel great when another person compliments them. You need to become that person who gives unexpected compliments.

Stop sharing your doom-and-gloom with the world

Each of you will have your own special manner and depth in the way you process this valuable information.   For those that follow my advice, your rewards will be carefree lives, newly attained health, minimized or obliterated stress, and transformation into a positive and optimistic person. Now, will it work for everyone? No – the facts are that some people enjoy complaining about their downfalls to others. Some people enjoy sharing doom-and-gloom with others, as this is what makes them feel comfortable. What is important for me is that a great number of readers who read this book will relate to what I am saying and will in fact take positive actions aimed at living a great life.

So, what is a great life? Ponder this statement for a minute: *Our lives are the sum of our memories. It is not the material possessions that we end up with or the amount of money that we have in the bank or the number of hours that we have spent at work.* No, if you were to strip a professional person of his/her suit, take away their cell phones, company car, job, and dropped them off in a secluded island, what they would have is their memories. No one can strip away your memories, except yourself.

Overcoming difficulties

You are the professional person who has been stripped of the business suit, the cell phone, the company car, the metropolitan lifestyle, the bank accounts, and now you sit at the beach on a secluded island with empty pockets. There is no one in sight. It is such a beautiful day. A mild breeze sways the mature palm trees near the beach area. You are in a state of disbelief. What happened to your smart cell phone? How will you contact your boss to tell him that you are running late? Will your project be turned in on time? None of this really matters right now because you have no way of communicating with the outside world.

Unbeknownst to you, new memories are being made. These are new memories of a beautiful beach with great weather and future opportunities. You see fish and know that you can eat. You see palm trees and see that you have shelter. You see a running stream and see that you have water. Positive memories are being made. These memories are in fact what will shape your future. *Accept the statement that our lives are the sum of our memories.* However, know that each day is an opportunity to start a new memory. Focus on what matters and ignore those events or memories that do not serve you well.

What about those of you who may not be able to shake off some bad memories? Well, the time has come for some hypnotherapy. Our brains are each wired differently. While some people can simply block out bad memories and replace those with new and positive memories, others may need a bit of help through hypnotherapy. Before beginning any hypnotherapy treatment, ask yourself some questions: "What do I want as part of this hypnotherapy? After the hypnotherapy treatment, how will I respond to stress and negative behavior or exposure? What process will I use to block out the distractions?

Testimonials

A person has smoked for seventeen years. He undergoes hypnotherapy and stops smoking in one day. A person who is a third degree black belt has had a life-long fear of spiders. He undergoes hypnotherapy and stops the fear after just one session. A person has been having ongoing nightmares about a car accident in which she suffered long-term injuries. She undergoes some hypnotherapy and after just one session is able to block out most negative thoughts about the accident. New and positive thoughts have now replaced prior negative thoughts. Although the above- mentioned results are not always typical, hypnotherapy can in fact help many people to pay attention on what is important versus being distracted by what is in the past and statistically unimportant.

The Blame Game

My parents were mean to me. Yeah, but now you are fifty years old and need to stop blaming them for the way you are. I was molested at a young age. I'm sorry to hear that you were molested, but each time you bring it up to complete strangers will be one more day that you are allowing this experience to define who you will become in your life. I was a victim of domestic violence ten years ago. Ok, but how much longer before you put those memories behind you and allow your new husband or boyfriend or wife or girlfriend the respect they deserve? I am a recovering alcoholic. Awesome, but it has been twenty years since your last drink and how much longer do you intend to be branded as a recovering alcoholic?

All of the above situations are of sample individuals who have endured pain and have overcome challenges. However, unless they do something to change their current thinking, the rest of their lives will be defined by the damaging events they endured in the past.

In order *to become happy, one must let go of anchors that may be holding us back.* Rather than keep re-hashing the past, one needs to create new memories that will in fact shape who they will become. Ask yourself: *How much more of my life am I willing to waste from the limited time I have left to live?* Don't be so lazy that you fail to process deeply what I am telling you. Reality check only comes but a few times in our lives. If you miss that bus too many times, you may be left all alone at the bus stop waiting for a new bus that will never arrive.

Are you willing to write a new storyline? Are you tired of living a mechanical life – almost as if you are repeating each daily activity over and over again? Are negative thoughts going around and around in your mind without any stop in sight? Similar to hypnotherapy, meditation offers an opportunity to step back as a way to get a different perspective on life matters.

Accept that you simply cannot change every event that happens to you in your life. What you can change is how you deal with each and every experience that comes your way.

Living a memorable life

Living a memorable life requires you to be the type of person who actively participates in positive life activities that are free from distractions. Learn to leave your cell phone in the car when you workout at the gym or buy groceries. Limit your time on the computer so that you do not ignore the fact that your children are growing up and need your wisdom and support. As you talk with other human beings, take your eyes off the cell phone and instead make eye contact with them so that you can have meaningful and memorable conversations.

Chapter 9: Tenacity, Resilience, and Survival Techniques

In terms of tenacity, you must focus your energies at pursuing your dreams. Whether you are a boy, a girl, a woman, or a man, if you are a capable and a hard working human being, you will be able to achieve your dreams. Yes, I realize that all of us have fear and such fear at times deters us from achieving our full potential. At the same time, God gave you eye sight for a specific reason. One of your eyes must focus on the opportunities, while the other eye focuses on the daily challenges of life. It is all a balancing act that must be learned and practiced.

Fear, strengths, opportunities, and challenges must all be balanced as each has a specific purpose in our lives. Without challenges, growth cannot occur. Without fear, opportunities would not present themselves. *Only by experiencing and embracing these conditions can you begin to attain a superior achievement level in your personal and professional life.*

Ambition and Resilience are Important Ingredients

While some people are inherently ambitious, such a personal trait can be learned or taught to others. *Ambition is in fact the driving force that creates a basis for resilience.* Why is it that some people overcome barriers and challenges in their lives while others crumple down and go away? The answer is resilience. Resilience is a unique trait that is created as a result of being exposed to overwhelming obstacles or challenges in light of little hope of survival. Very few human beings can say that taking risks comes easily to them. If they do, it is simply a routine to experience such risks and oftentimes these are not considered challenges.

Take for example a military fighter pilot who is used to flying dangerous missions. Such a pilot expects to get attacked and has received proper training to respond to such attacks. However, a commercial airline pilot who does not expect to be attacked would not be prepared for such an incident. Such was the case of the American commercial airline pilot who had just taken off from an airport near the Hudson River. As the plane's nose was still aimed high, both plane engines stalled and he had to make an immediate decision on where he could safely land the plane. Luckily, he had previous military experience that allowed him to glide the plane safely into the Hudson River. All passengers survived and he was hailed a hero.

Review the same scenario and ask yourself what if the pilot had decided to make a U-turn and return to the airport for an emergency landing on hard ground? What if during such landing many passengers were injured and even killed? What would happen then? Well, the pilot's actions would be investigated and he would be prosecuted if it was found that his actions violated policy or the safety of his passengers. Such investigation may in fact land him in jail. So, from this example we can see that *in life, your choices are always half-chanced.* Half the time you may be right and the other half you may be wrong. One day you are a hero and the next day you can become a convicted criminal due to circumstances beyond your control.

Life then involves a series of survival techniques. Such survival techniques must begin with your conscious decision to take care of your personal needs first, before you are able to take care of other's needs.   If you have some time, read about Maslow's Hierarchy of needs. Our bodies have specific needs that must be met so that we can be happy and feel fulfilled. Now, these must be realistic needs – not exaggerated needs like: I want to be a millionaire now or, tomorrow I expect to have $200,000 in my savings account.

While some who read this may say: "Ah, wait a minute, I was able to make that happen. Why shouldn't others do the same?" *The simple answer for this question is that personal goals must be specific to each individual and their circumstances.* A person with stage four terminal cancers may have more significant life goals compared to a fully healthy young person who has an entire future ahead of them. The key is that survival is specific to each individual. Each individual must have a survival plan that will meet her/his needs at various stages of their lives.

Self-Empowerment

Empower yourself to talk about life opportunities. Everyone has an opinion and you always have a choice on which opinion you listen to and eventually adopt. Information in life is so distorted that many don't know what works or what doesn't work. Persons who often take many prescription medications often arrive at a point that they do not know what is working and what is not working. As such, a cleansing process must occur where they must stop what they are doing and begin at a new "Fresh Start" in their life race."

Practice stopping others who want to tell you about doom and gloom in their lives. Learn to tell them: "You are wasting your time talking about things that happened in the past. The only way you will be happy and get a new perspective in life is to begin talking positive and not wasting your time with negative conversation." Rude? No. Awkward? Maybe. But, you must learn to tell others this or they will likely impair your progress into a happiness state of mind.

Be cautious on what information you adopt once you have created a new "Start" point in your life. The main reason for this is that there are those people out there who are waiting for the right moment to take advantage of someone like you. Whether it is religion, a business idea, an investment idea, a nutrition idea, a multi-level scam, a doctor's prescription, such representatives always have something to gain by convincing you that what they are selling is exactly what you and others need.

Learn to say: "No, Thank you." And walk away.

Stop and question the necessity for any product or belief that is being offered to you. *What is the validity and value to you directly?* What are the consequences if you chose to accept or buy into the concept? Will it help or hurt you in the short and long-term? Have you read or looked at information on both sides? Information is power, but be careful where such information is coming from. Those with influence will always try to convert those who lack such a capacity level. Don't become a sheep.

Each of us is a soldier in life and each day requires us to abide by survival techniques. Food, shelter, and clothing are your three main needs. But, did you know that while you can go without food for a long period of time, shelter must be obtained early on or you will not make it?

We read about how some people who were out hiking and got lost. Days, and weeks go by. After some time, the news reports on such survival stories. Survival experts will tell you that if you get lost, set your priorities in finding a base camp where you will have shelter. A cave, or a makeshift shack all provide shelter from the elements and can be used to your survival benefit. Making a fire which will provide warmth and finding food will be next on your list. Even if you can't find food, you will need to return to your shelter before dark. These are human instincts, which are built into our DNA.

Applying survival techniques in everyday life

If we are to apply such survival techniques to our urban or rural way of living, we must abide by all natural principles. Doing so is one of the fast track ways we are going to overcome happiness barriers and other obstacles in our lives. A methodical and oftentimes natural plan must be developed and implemented if you are to move from your current situation to a more ideal situation.

Start Building Your Fort

The first pig built a straw house only to find that the wind blew it away. The second pig built a wood/pallets house only to find out that the wind and a mean wolf blew it away. Only the oldest and wisest pig was smart enough to build a house made of bricks. Such design knowledge took into consideration the nature's elements as well as enemies that would eventually come and try to make illegal entry into the pig's home. Well, you know what? Life is full of wolves who are constantly trying to gain ground around you. You must constantly take protective steps, which are aimed at seeking adequate shelter and protection from such enemies. Failure to do so, will cause you to become victims of the system.

Chapter 10: Music, Misery, Anti-Aging, Antioxidants and the Obstacle Course

The world is a playground full of possibilities. We all know this but somehow between childhood and now, many seemed to have forgotten what it means to do what is fun and avoid that which causes pain.

With possibilities, we understand that distractions are always present. Yes, and some of those distractions at times can consume our minds and cause us some pain. Please know that growing pains are good for the mind and soul. However, any un-natural pain that causes constant sadness and depression is bad for the mind and soul and should be avoided or removed from your life.

Take a look at your current life library and see what needs to be discarded. Make some piles and label them: Sell, Keep, Not sure. Get rid of the Sell and Not sure piles. *Uncertainty is not good when positive change is waiting for you.*

Go through the Keep pile and sort out what you still need to throw away. Keep only that which warms your soul with positive energy. Discard everything that you know is damaging to your body and soul. Remove all library items that remind you of bad places in your life. You become that which you attract and being constantly sad or reminded of negative experiences only brings those back into your life.

A smell, a place, or songs can take us to places we no longer wish to visit. Recognize this. *Harness the power of feeding your body with only those experiences, which bring you joy.* They say that too much joy is well... too much. However, I disagree with this statement. Joy is in itself good for the body and soul. One cannot ever have too much joy in their lives.

Makes Me Feel Like Dancing

What music makes you feel like dancing? What beats move your soul? People listen to music for a variety of reasons. It makes you feel happy, it makes you feel sad, it makes you feel adventurous, it makes you think, ponder, and contemplate. Music has such a powerful effect on the human soul. Now – listening to the right music matters because each song brings with it certain outcomes.

A person who is ready to do a weight lifting workout may want some heart pounding music on as she or he prepares for their workout. A person who is ready to begin meditating will listen to soothing music with natural sounds such as waterfalls, the sound of wind or ocean glistening in the background. The middle ground are songs that make you feel loved, sad, depressed, or angry. Yes – music does in fact take control of your mind. That is – if you let it.

You have to recognize the real power of music and use it to create positive change in your life. Heavy metal music will not calm your mind if your mind seeks peace, quiet, and stillness. Rock and roll music will not help your meditation exercises.

Classical music? Well, the jury is still out on that one. I want you to think about what type of music you have been listening to. If you are sad as a result of a broken relationship, the last thing you want to do is listen to love songs. The worst thing you can do is to listen to those love songs that remind you of the person who created so much sadness or depression in your life.

Music is situational and you must harness its power to affect the Happiness Yoga Power of Rehearsal into your life. Garbage in – garbage out. Positive in – positive out. Find that music which inspires you. Find that music which relaxes you. Find that music which slows life down so that you can clearly see what is taking place. *Stop listening to music which you know is damaging your soul.* Stop listening to music that you know is making you feel sad, depressed, or angry. Yes, get rid of that bad music completely. Create playlists in your I-pod or other music player that are labeled: Motivational, Positive, meditating, Adventurous, Inspiring, and Mind building. Delete all songs, which brings you negative feelings into your body. At first, changing your music habits may take some work and a bit of pain. But, soon you will begin to feel your body come in tune with nature.

Body and Earth's Electrical Current

There is an electrical current running through the earth that is the same frequency as the electrical current running in your body. You will notice that once you remove bad music and other similar influences from your life, that electrical current will flow unobstructed. You will become happier. You will feel healthier. You will start to notice things around you that you had never noticed. Happiness is possible.

More on the electrical current or magnetic therapy can be found by researching *Medithera mats.* Learn about the earth's magnetic pulse and how you can use this to program your body to become healthy and happy. There are a number of these devices out there and it is best for you to research each of them to see which one meets your needs. BioMat: Contains different crystals, jade, amethyst, etc. It uses different wavelengths of far infrared waves and it heats up. It can be programmed for various amounts of heat and time. This device has won several awards. There are various healing programs within these machines. Some devices can be rented before purchase. There are beds with magnets embedded in them. The ultimate focus is to get your body in tune with its own accurate frequency.

Other than BioMats, there are other sheets of silver thread that is woven into the fabric. These sheets have a wire that you plug into the ground and it syncs to the frequency of the earth. Their companies have conducted studies on their products. These studies show an improvement in the body's healing power.

No one product offers a "Cure-all" for all conditions. However, your goal is to pick the best product that will work for your situation. The mere availability of these products affords you choices that you may not have known existed before reading this book.

Antioxidants and Anti-Aging

Antioxidants are protective molecules that can be found in a number of digestible foods. These are the equivalent of millions of tiny soldiers within your body that help fight a number of common diseases. Where can these be found? Antioxidants are found in a number of natural fruits and vegetables. A list of these fruits and vegetables will be included at the end of this section.

Health or Wealth? Or... Both?

A wealthy man asked his son who was leaving for college what car he wanted to buy. The son thought about it for a few days and then returned with his request. "Dad, I don't want a car, instead, can you buy me a comfortable pillow top mattress?" The father was a bit confused and asked his son why. The son replied that he could use public transportation and friend's cars for rides while he was attending college. However, he knew that he would be getting a great night's sleep if he had a great quality mattress to return to at the end of a stressful day.

A rich man was asked to choose between his health and his fortune. He chose health. Why? If he has health, he knows that he can find new wealth. Plus, if we are not healthy, it is difficult to be happy. If we are not healthy, our bodies are susceptible to various cancers. As we get older we hear about a number of our friends and family who have been diagnosed with various types of cancer. If we accept that cancer is a reality, we must take preventative steps against allowing it to enter our bodies.

So, can we prevent cancer from entering our bodies? Yes. However, it takes a realistic and preventative attitude coupled with action steps to make this happen. The preventative attitude I am referring to here is that you must become aware and understand your body's own level of antioxidants. This level can be tested using a Biophotonic scanner.

You need antioxidants to protect your DNA from free radical and harmful chemicals that are absorbed by your body from a number of common exposures. Exposures to smog, personal injuries, trauma, cigarette smoke, chemical pollution, medications, radiation, poorly cooked food, stress, and fried foods all bring free radical and other toxin genes such as Mercury into our bodies.

Pharmanex's Biophotonic scanner uses a 90 seconds non-invasive procedure to measure the skin's level of antioxidants. This level equates to the same level of antioxidants that are present in your body. Using color code bars, this device measures a person's Carotenoid Scores. Anyone who scores 50,000 and above has the optimum level of antioxidants in their bodies. This score would be the equivalent of an 'A' Grade.

'B' grade persons score in the 40,000 to 49,000 range. 'C' grade persons score in the 30,000 to 39,000 range. 'D' grade persons score in the 20,000 to 29,000 range. Lastly, 'E' grade persons are those who score in the 10, 000 to 19,000 range. Persons who score in the low C, D, & E levels should learn what they can do to raise their body's antioxidants' level.

Organic foods contain a higher level of antioxidants.

Foods containing a high level of antioxidants:

Brussel Sprouts
Broccoli
Raspberries
Tomatoes
Coffee (without cream or sugar)
Roasted Peanuts
Tea (without milk)
Parsley
Flax Seed
Kale
Spinach
Chicory
Swiss Chard
Red Cabbage
Kumquats

Antioxidant vegetables should be steamed and not boiled.

Pharmanex's dietary supplements such as LifePak Nano allows the body to absorb higher levels of antioxidants. You can also drink smoothies that include Kale, Carrots, Apple Banana, Pears, Strawberries, Raspberries, Flax Seed, Peaches, or Nectarines.

In terms of anti-aging, a number of health professionals recommend that you take supplements such as Omega-3 fats, and perform moderate exercise so as to reduce frailty and improve your body's core strength. Eating a healthy diet such as the antioxidant vegetables and fruits mentioned in this chapter will allow you stay happy, look young and stay younger longer.

To read more about this topic, look up the antioxidant *Glutathione.* The purpose of this antioxidant is that it recycles all of the antioxidants in a person's body. Research Doctor Mark Hyman, M.D. to learn more about Glutathione.

Misery Loves Company

Comedian Russell Peters once said that the very worst thing that could happen to a comedian is to achieve complete happiness. When he was asked to clarify, he explained that when a comedian is happy, he or she has nothing to complain about. On the other hand, when a comedian is miserable, he seems to connect better with the audience. By communicating misery stories to others, we tend to connect with the wider audience as many of them are enduring daily difficulties in their lives.

If you find this hard to believe, try this with your friends or co-workers. For three weeks you arrive at work. Whenever a friend or co-worker asks how you are doing, tell them about all of your difficulties in life: Your old car broke down, you ran out of gas, you are having relationship problems with your boyfriend, girlfriend, wife, husband, etc. You don't like your job. A friend refused to help you. Your boyfriend or girlfriend left you. You haven't been feeling well, etc. Watch and learn how people react when you tell them about your misery. Most often they will: Listen with a sympathetic ear. They will offer you advice or support. They will feel sorry for you and suggest a solution. They will check up on you to see how you are doing. They will seek out help for you in your problem areas or they will simply avoid you after labeling you a negative person.

On the opposite side of this experiment: Provide your co-workers or friends with short neutral answers when they ask how you are doing. Do this for several weeks. Your replies should be something like: "I'm good thank you" and walk away. "Nothing new in my life and then walk away." "Thanks for asking but nothing interesting to report" and then walk away. Once you have neutralized your audience of friends and co-workers… try a third and different approach.

For at least three weeks… whenever anyone asks you how you are doing, you reply: "Wonderful, couldn't be better" or "My life is the best it could be" or, "I have the best relationship in the world and no complaints from me" or "I feel healthy and have never felt any better. Each time you do this, pause for a few seconds after your response and then walk away. What you will find at the end of your experiment is that whenever you tell people that your life is great, perfect, trouble-free, complaint-free, fulfilled, etc., people's replies will be shorter and at times abrupt.

The majority of the population in our lives actually thrives on conflict and if you remove the conflict away from the conversation, then you remove the very "misery" that they want to hear, want to comment on, want to discuss, or offer their own advice. In addition, the positive responses you adopt will end office gossip, which often involves telling others about the turmoil in one's life. Believe me that those people who are addicted to soap operas are in fact our co-workers, our friends, and our family members.

Obstacle Course

How much soul-searching have you done lately? People usually say: "Lately I have done a lot of soul searching and…" How would you complete that phrase? Would it say "…and I am really happy at the way my life is heading" or, "…and I am tired of the way my life has been going?" The power of choice is indeed one that involves a number of obstacles. So, let's take you to the obstacle course.

The day you arrive at the obstacle course everything seems strange. You look at the number of obstacles that have been laid out in this open area. Wow! You think to yourself. How am I supposed to complete all of these challenges? One obstacle is a huge wall that appears to be six stories tall. The other obstacle requires you to maneuver a tricky obstacle course that runs through mud puddles, dirt holes, small mountains of dirt, balancing bars, sway ropes, and a water hole. Your doubts overcome you. You begin to get nervous and your internal voice questions your ability to conquer all of these challenges.

As you quietly observe the obstacle course, other participants arrive. Some of these people are tall, short, skinny, or overweight. Some are obviously strong and athletic while others are of average build. You scan the audience possibly trying to find one of the participants that looks somewhat like you. You see a couple of people that could match, but each of the persons has unique differences that are surely not identical to you. You shake your head and begin to realize that you will participate in this event alone and strive to do your best.

The instructor arrives, yet – you can't see him. It's merely a stern voice talking to everyone in this group. The voice welcomes everyone and is calming as it explains that the object is not to get the best time or to outperform other participants but to simply complete the course at your own pace. "Take your time and plan your actions accordingly" the voice says. "Scan and assess your surroundings. Know your limitations. Push those limitations to new heights. Caution is advisable but it should not hinder your success. Rather, it will help you during the times when you feel like giving up. You and only you can get through this course. While other participants may give you advice, it will be up to you to either accept, or ignore such advice. Remember that some participants are actually here to see you fail. If you realize that good and evil are always present, you will be successful and achieve happiness. Recognize fear but learn to fight through it. This concludes my introduction. You may now begin the challenge course." Although the voice disappears, you still feel that it is there with you.

You begin the course and it seems very strange and uncomfortable at first. Yet, you learn to master each obstacle or part of the course. Every once in a while, you fall down. It hurts to fall down. As you get back up, you assess why you fell down. You don't want to make the same mistakes twice. You look around and see others fall. While some participants are helping others, you see that some of the participants are actually sitting on top of others who have fallen down. You are surprised, but busy with your own challenges.

You look ahead and notice that other participants are actually holding some participants back intentionally. Some of the mean participants are pushing their colleagues off the obstacle course. They actually enjoy seeing people fall. They actually enjoy misery. You know this is not you. You continue through the obstacle course ignoring the distractions. You realize there is sadness and hurtful behavior taking place in the obstacle course, yet you choose to stay happy and work through your challenges.

Towards the end of the obstacle course you look up and realize. *You realize that the obstacle course was your Life.* The obstacle course is almost over and you force yourself to slow down. The very event you began looking to finish is now changed. You realize that you have to slow down as you are living on borrowed time. You learn to slow or completely stop so that you can hear the sound of stillness. You meditate. You eat right. You choose your best friends for your new team. You learn to appreciate that which has been given you and ignore that which you cannot control. From this point on you will decide how to proceed in your obstacle course.

Life is half-chanced so always choose that which makes you happy, fulfilled, appreciated, and loved.

Closing Remarks

This book is one of many books about happiness. Each of those dedicated authors sought out to help you in your quest to find happiness. While you may not agree with everything that is presented in these books, you must recognize that the decision to become happy has been and will always rest with you. *You have the power to become happy.* You have the power to erase bad memories and replace them with new positive memories. You have the ability to focus your mind on that which is positive and encouraging. Don't simply live your life by default. Search for and find that which allows you to operate in a positive mindset. Enjoy all that life is. Treasure every experience, as each moment is a gift.

Learn to live a life that is abundant in happiness. This Yoga Power of Rehearsal book sought to free your mind from those deeply rooted beliefs that had been keeping you in sadness for far too long. *Your mind has been set free.* You have been given the proper tools and these are now available for your use within your mind. Go out and rehearse those very actions that will bring you a new level of happiness.

The person you were has changed. Those persons in your past have changed. Past situations have changed. *In fact, those very memories of past events are only kept alive in your mind by you.* Release those memories. Release the pain and free up your mind so that it will allow you to be the person you have always intended to be.

You are now on your path towards gratitude and happiness. *Allow a consistent push to grow your awareness* as you move forward in your new life. Once your eyes open from a night's sleep, be thankful and grateful that you are alive. Jump out of bed and begin your day. This is your Gift!

There will be deaths, divorces, separations, breakups, loss of jobs, and other disappointments in life. However, *don't lose sight of your internal purpose focus.* Your main focus should be to adapt to and experience those very things that allow your journey to be and stay positive.

What is your own mystical calling? Learn not to return to the past. You may look in the rear view mirror every once in a while to remind yourself where you have been, yet – returning there should never be an option. Start building your new mystical fort today. Use the foundational strategies mentioned in this book and just do it!

You have your bags packed but you don't need them. What baggage have you accumulated that needs to be discarded? Only you can answer this question. Get away from those archaic anchors or deeply rooted beliefs that are blocking your true positive spirit. *Find that fuel that moves you closer to your dreams.* Don't allow any distractions to derail you from your intended purpose.

If you want to stay transformed, be and stay committed towards this transformation. Be the role model for others who are also seeking their happiness. Be the person who others admire and seek out for inspiration.

When you are all alone with yourself, you can actually find who you are. This is perfectly normal. *Don't allow yourself to become lost.* Instead, find the treasure of who you are and what you can do with this amazing gift that we call Life.

There is a story that needs to be written. That story will be written by the new you.

Dr. Bryan Silva, Ph.D.

The End